Type 2 Diabetes
BASICS

Third Edition

Patti Rickheim, MS, RN, CDE

Jill Flader, MS, RD, LD, CDE

with Karol M. Carstensen

Revision Team

Jill Flader, MS, RD, LD, CDE

Nancy Cooper, RD, LD, CDE

David Randal, PsyD, LP, CDE

International Diabetes Center

Park Nicollet

Type 2 Diabetes BASICS is the learner guide for a diabetes education program by the same name. The book is organized in sections that coincide with the four sessions of the program, which is typically taught by nurses and dietitians who are certified diabetes educators (CDE).

Readers may use this book outside of the program format. However, we strongly advise all people with diabetes to seek appropriate medical care and diabetes education from trained healthcare professionals.

International Diabetes Center
3800 Park Nicollet Boulevard
Minneapolis, MN 55416-2699
internationaldiabetescenter.com

Quantity discounts and customizations are available. For information or to order, please call 1-888-637-2675 or log on to idcpublishing.com.

This publication is intended for informational purposes only and cannot serve as a substitute for the care provided by a licensed physician or health care provider. Readers are advised to seek medical guidance before making any changes in self-care practices or medical therapies. Neither can this publication serve as a substitute for the policies and protocols agreed to and followed by medical institutions. Health care providers wishing to adopt all or part of the information provided herein for clinical practice are advised to seek approval from appropriate authorities in their institutions.

Managing Editor: Pat Boland
Editor: Corrine Casanova
Production Manager: Lisa Feder
Design and Text Production: Christopher Bennett
Illustrations: John Bush

Printed in the United States of America

15 14 13 12   3 4 5 6

Acknowledgments

The authors would like to thank the Type 2 Diabetes BASICS team at International Diabetes Center, Minneapolis, MN, for their commitment to the program and to our patients.

Richard M. Bergenstal, MD

Kristin Carlson, RD, LD, CDE

Robert M. Cuddihy, MD

Janet Davidson, BSN, RN, CDE

Nancy Destache, BSN, RN, CDE

Mary Droogsma, RN, CDE

Paula Ekerholm, MS, RD, LD, CDE

Colleen Fischer, RD, LD, CDE

Maureen Kayser, BSN, RN, CDE

Deanne Kendhammer, RN, CDE

Melissa Klohn, RD, LD, CDE

Julie Kunz, RD, LD, CDE

Kristin Kunzman, PysD, LP

Mamie Lausch, MS, RN, RD, CDE

Janet Lima, MPH, RN, CDE

Dianna Martin, RN

Ronica Norton, BSN, RN, CDE

Shannon Perron, RD, LD, CDE

Margaret Powers, PhD, RD, CDE

Diane Reader, RD, LD, CDE

Kathleen Reynolds, RN, CDE

Debra Schiesl, BSN, RN, CDE

Sue Sorensen, RD, LD, CDE

Anna Vannelli, RD, LD, CDE

Nancy Waldbillig, RD, LD, CDE

Mary Ziotas Zacharatos, RD, LD, CDE

Table of Contents

Introduction

Nearly 24 million people in the United States have diabetes. That number doesn't include the 57 million people who have prediabetes. No matter how much or little you know about diabetes, this book can help.

This book is divided into four sections and will provide a good framework for what you need to know about diabetes. It will describe what diabetes is and the different ways to treat it. You will discover how food, activity, and stress affect diabetes. You will also learn how to test your blood glucose (sugar). You will do this with the help of your diabetes care team.

Your diabetes care team consists of you (the most important member), your physician, physician assistant, nurse practitioner, registered nurse, registered dietitian, psychologist, social worker, and pharmacist. Professionals who have passed the National Certification Exam are Certified Diabetes Educators (CDE).

Although diabetes is a chronic condition, millions of people live full, happy lives while managing their diabetes. You can too.

Welcome

In this session, you will:

- Gain an understanding of diabetes and what causes it
- Learn how diabetes is treated and the goals of treatment
- Learn why, how, and when to test your glucose
- Learn how carbohydrate affects your glucose
- Receive a personal food plan and learn how to count carbohydrates
- Discover how physical activity enhances glucose control and overall health
- Begin to gain confidence in your ability to manage diabetes

What Is Diabetes?

Diabetes means that your blood glucose, or blood sugar, is too high. When food is digested, much of it changes into glucose (or sugar) in your blood. Glucose is fuel for your body. Your bloodstream carries the glucose to your cells, which use it for energy.

Beta cells in your pancreas make insulin to help glucose get into cells. Insulin attaches to each cell and lets glucose inside.

Sometimes, your body can't make enough insulin or your cells "resist" insulin and glucose can't enter your cells. When this happens, glucose levels in your blood rise. This is diabetes.

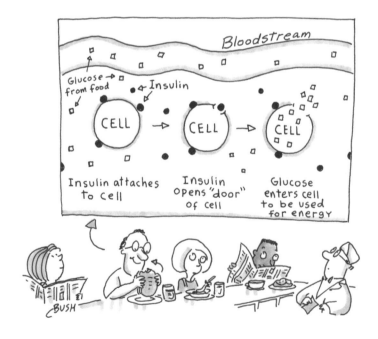

Types of Diabetes

There are three types of diabetes. Each type happens for a different reason. No type of diabetes is worse. All three cause high glucose levels.

Type 2 Diabetes

In type 2 diabetes, your body can't use insulin properly. It "resists" the action of insulin. It is difficult for glucose to get into your body's cells, so it stays in your blood. Over time, your pancreas makes less insulin. This is why people who have type 2 diabetes may need to take diabetes pills and/or insulin. Type 2 diabetes is most common in adults. However, it's becoming more common in children.

Type 1 Diabetes

In type 1 diabetes, your body can't make insulin. Type 1 diabetes can happen at any age, although usually it occurs in children and young adults under age 30. If you have type 1 diabetes, you need to take insulin every day because your pancreas doesn't produce it.

Gestational Diabetes

Women need extra insulin when they are pregnant because of hormonal changes. Some women can't make more insulin. Their glucose levels go up, and they develop gestational diabetes. A woman's glucose usually returns to normal after her baby is born. However, her chances of developing type 2 diabetes later on are higher.

Diabetes Diagnosis, Risk Factors, and Symptoms

Diagnosis

Diabetes is diagnosed by measuring the level of glucose in your blood. The following tests are used for diagnosis:

- An **A1C test** measures your average glucose level over the last two to three months. This laboratory test can be done at any time of day. (See page 14 for more about the A1C test.)

- A **fasting glucose test** measures your glucose level when you've had nothing to eat or drink (except water) for at least eight hours.

- A **random glucose test** can be used to measure your glucose level at any time of day.

- An **oral glucose tolerance test (OGTT)** measures your glucose level when you've had nothing to eat or drink (except water) for at least eight hours, and again two hours after you drink a sweetened beverage.

An elevated test result often needs to be repeated on a separate day to confirm the diagnosis of diabetes.

Diagnosis	A1C	Fasting Glucose	Random Glucose*	2-hour OGTT
Diabetes	6.5% or higher	126 mg/dL or higher	200 mg/dL or higher with symptoms	200 mg/dL or higher
Prediabetes	5.7–6.4%	100–125 mg/dL		140–199 mg/dL

* Random glucose test cannot be used to diagnose prediabetes.

Prediabetes

When glucose is higher than normal, but not high enough to be diabetes, it is called prediabetes. If you have prediabetes, you are at higher risk for developing type 2 diabetes. Studies show that many people with prediabetes go on to develop diabetes within 10 years. However, there are steps you can take to delay or possibly prevent this from happening.

Being overweight can make your body resistant to the action of insulin. Losing weight and being more active can help your body respond better to insulin. Research shows that if you lose as few as 10 to 15 pounds and get at least 150 minutes of physical activity each week, you may be able to reduce your risk for developing type 2 diabetes by more than *half*.

No matter what your diagnosis is, the idea is to control your glucose level. Doing this now will help you to stay healthy.

Type 2 Diabetes Risk Factors

Diabetes risk factors fall into three categories: genetic, personal health history, and lifestyle.

Genetic and some personal health history factors, such as a family history of diabetes or a personal history of diabetes during pregnancy, cannot be changed.

Lifestyle factors, such as being inactive or smoking, can be changed. Making these changes can improve other risk factors such as high blood pressure or cholesterol. Positive changes in these areas can also reduce the risk of developing diabetes.

Answer the questions on page 9. This may help you understand your diagnosis. It will also show you areas that you may want to work on. Ask your family members to answer the questions, too. They are at risk for diabetes because they have a family history.

The physical activity and nutrition recommendations in this book support a healthy lifestyle. Following them will help people with diabetes, those with prediabetes, and those at risk for diabetes. In fact, everyone can benefit, so encourage your family to get involved, too.

What Are Your Risk Factors for Type 2 Diabetes?

Answer the following questions.

Yes : No

☐ : ☐   Are you overweight?

☐ : ☐   Do you smoke?

☐ : ☐   Does someone in your family have diabetes?

☐ : ☐   Are you inactive?

☐ : ☐   Are you African American, Native American, Hispanic or Latino, Asian, Alaska Native, Native Hawaiian, or a Pacific Islander?

☐ : ☐   Has your glucose level ever been high?

☐ : ☐   Have you had diabetes during pregnancy or a baby weighing more than 9 pounds at birth?

☐ : ☐   Do you have heart or blood vessel disease?

☐ : ☐   Do you have high blood pressure?

☐ : ☐   Do you have abnormal blood cholesterol or triglycerides?

☐ : ☐   Have you ever had polycystic ovary syndrome?

☐ : ☐   Do you have dark velvety patches of skin (acanthosis nigricans) on the back of your neck, in your armpits, on your elbows, or anywhere else on your body?

"Yes" answers show your risk factors for type 2 diabetes. If you have questions, talk with your care team.

Diabetes Symptoms

Some people have many symptoms. Some have none at all and find it hard to believe the diagnosis. Certain symptoms are more common with type 2 diabetes. Others are more common with type 1 diabetes. However, any symptoms shown in the table below can happen with either type of diabetes.

Type 2 Diabetes	Type 1 Diabetes
Fatigue	Frequent urination
Blurred vision	Increased thirst
Cuts and sores that don't heal	Increased hunger
Dry, itchy skin	Unexplained weight loss
Infections (or the same infection keeps coming back)	
Numbness and tingling in hands, legs, or feet	

Most diabetes symptoms clear up with treatment. In fact, it's only after they are gone that many people recognize that they had symptoms in the first place. For example, many people have more energy after beginning treatment. They just didn't realize that the tiredness they felt before being diagnosed was because of high glucose levels.

Diabetes Complications

When your glucose levels are regularly high, it can lead to other health problems. This doesn't happen overnight. There are things you can do. Taking care of your diabetes can help prevent, delay, or slow this process.

The chart below shows areas of the body that may have complications from diabetes.

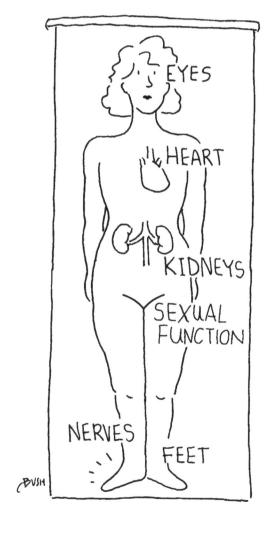

Type 2 Diabetes Treatment

The goals of diabetes treatment are to help you:

- Keep your glucose levels in target

- Keep your blood pressure and cholesterol levels in target

- Balance your diabetes treatment plan with your daily life

- Prevent, delay, or slow the progression of health problems caused by diabetes

- Feel better every day

A food plan and regular physical activity are part of every diabetes treatment plan. Diabetes medications may be needed too. These may include diabetes pills or insulin injections. A new type of injection that helps the body make more insulin is also available. All of these medications help to lower glucose. A combination of them may be needed. Each of the individual medications is described on pages 108–110 in the *Appendix*.

How Different Diabetes Medications Work

- Help the pancreas release more insulin

- Help the body use insulin better

- Make the liver release less glucose

- Slow down the absorption of carbohydrate

- Help pancreas cells work better

- Gives body extra insulin

Pills work to lower glucose in different ways. The type and dose of pill depends on your glucose levels. More than one type of pill may be needed.

Sometimes pills aren't enough to lower glucose. A long-acting insulin called a "background" insulin may be added. An injection once a day provides extra insulin all day long. You will still need to take diabetes pills during the day.

Another type of injected medicine can help your pancreas make more insulin when you eat. Some people find it helps them eat less at meals and may lead to weight loss.

The best treatment plan is the one that keeps your glucose level in control. Some people need to take pills or insulin right away when they are diagnosed with diabetes. Others don't. Treatment plans change over time (see below).

Diabetes Treatment Options

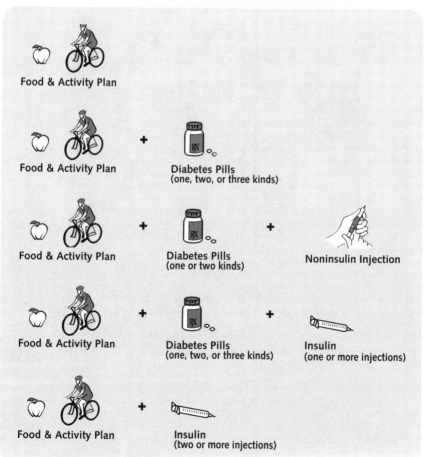

Food & Activity Plan

Food & Activity Plan + Diabetes Pills (one, two, or three kinds)

Food & Activity Plan + Diabetes Pills (one or two kinds) + Noninsulin Injection

Food & Activity Plan + Diabetes Pills (one, two, or three kinds) + Insulin (one or more injections)

Food & Activity Plan + Insulin (two or more injections)

The A1C Test

A1C is a laboratory blood test that shows your average glucose level over the last two to three months. It lets you know how well your diabetes treatment is working.

A1C measures the amount of glucose attached to your hemoglobin. Red blood cells contain hemoglobin that carries oxygen to your body's tissues. When glucose is high, more sticks to your hemoglobin. A normal A1C is about 4% to 6%.

The A1C target for many people who have diabetes is less than 7%.*

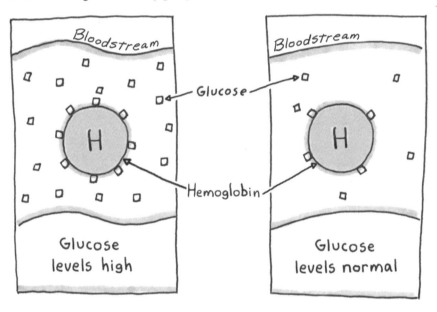

Your care team will work with you to develop a treatment plan to help reach your target. It may take a few months to reach. Any improvement in A1C is a step toward better health. An A1C is usually scheduled three to four times a year.

* Less stringent A1C goals are appropriate for some people. Check with your care team for your individual target.

Testing Your Blood Glucose

Testing your glucose is another important way to see if your diabetes is in control. This tells you what your glucose level is at the very moment you test.

You do this test yourself using a glucose meter. Keep a record of your test results in your diabetes record book.

Your test results help you and your care team to:

- See how well your treatment plan is working

- Decide what changes you may need to make

- See how these changes affect your glucose levels

When to Test Your Glucose

To start out, it is best to do three tests each day at these times:

- Before breakfast

- Before your main meal

- Two hours after the start of your main meal

Follow this schedule for the next two weeks. Write your test results in your diabetes record book. After this, you may be able to test less often.

Your Glucose Targets

Keeping your glucose level in target helps you manage your diabetes better. Before you can aim for a target, you need to know what your target is. The following table shows the recommended glucose targets depending on the time of your glucose test.

Your care team may give you different targets, depending on your personal health needs. If so, write them in the space provided below.

Test Time	Diabetes Target (mg/dL)	My Target	No Diabetes/ Prediabetes (mg/dL)
Before a meal	70–120		Less than 100
2 hours after the start of a meal	Less than 160		Less than 140

Your glucose level naturally goes up after you eat. That happens to everyone. Pay attention to how much it goes up.

Check your results against your targets. Sometimes your glucose level will be out of target. They don't have to be perfect. Work toward having at least half (50%) of all your test results in target at each of the times you test.

Sample Record Book

Date	Night BG	BREAKFAST BG	BREAKFAST Med	BG	LUNCH BG	LUNCH Med	BG	EVENING MEAL BG	EVENING MEAL Med	BG	BEDTIME BG	BEDTIME Med
6-5		159	Metformin 500mg					138	Metformin 500mg	181		
6-6		136						94		138		
6-7		126						169		199		

16

Glucose Test Results and Your A1C

Your A1C and your daily glucose test results are linked. When at least half (50%) of your tests are in target overall, your A1C usually will be in target too. The following table shows how these two numbers relate. For example, if at least half of your glucose test numbers are between 210 and 245, your A1C will be about 9%.

A1C Value
(Target is less than 7%)

Daily Glucose Testing Average
(Goal is to have half or more tests in target)

A1C Value	Daily Glucose Testing Average
4%	50–80
5%	80–115
6%	115–150
7%	150–180
8%	180–210
9%	210–245
10%	245–280
11%	280–310
12%	310–345
13%	345 or greater

Daily glucose tests help determine if you need to make any adjustments to your treatment plan, and where they need to be made. If your daily glucose test numbers are getting better, then your next A1C value will be better too.

Glucose Meters

Glucose meters are battery operated devices. They "read" your glucose level from a very small drop of blood. The meter displays the result on a small screen.

To use most meters, you insert a test strip into the meter. Then you poke your finger with a lancet and apply a small drop of blood to the strip. The strip has chemicals in it that react with the blood. This allows the meter to get a reading.

Most meters require a blood sample from a finger poke. Some will accept blood from a small poke on your forearm or another site on your body. Your care team will help you choose the right meter for you.

Testing may seem hard at first, but it will get easier as time goes on.

Sharps Disposal

Lancets and syringe needles are called *sharps*. Do not throw them in the trash. They need to be placed in a special sharps container to avoid injuring other people. Most drug stores or pharmacies sell sharps containers. Some will also take the container once it is full and dispose of it.

If your pharmacy doesn't take used sharps, contact your city, county, or state health department about programs in your area for collecting them.

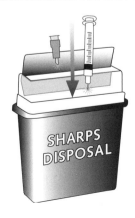

How to Test Your Glucose

No matter what brand of meter you have, follow these general guidelines when you test your glucose.*

1. Wash hands with soap and warm water or use an alcohol wipe. (Avoid hand sanitizers.) Dry hands well.

2. Shake arm down to get more blood into fingertips.

3. Put a test strip into meter (see your meter instructions).

4. Poke the side of fingertip with lancing device.

5. Gently rub or massage the area until a drop of blood appears.

6. Apply blood drop to test strip.

7. Wait for meter to show result.

8. Record result in diabetes record book.

9. Dispose of lancet properly.

* Some meters can test blood from the forearm or other areas. However, avoid using these sites within two hours of a meal or when you suspect a low glucose.

Each time you test, use a new lancet. Alternate among all ten fingers. If you have questions about your meter, call the toll-free number on the meter.

Your Diabetes Food Plan

Much of the food you eat is broken down and turned into glucose. That is why a food plan is an important part of your diabetes treatment. Your dietitian will work with you to create a food plan that is right for you.

Your food plan is based on:

- What, when, and how much you like to eat
- Your lifestyle, including activity level
- Your health needs
- Your weight goal

You don't have to eat special foods. There is no strict diabetes diet. You can still enjoy the foods you like—just in moderation. A food plan typically includes three meals a day. It may also include snacks.

When you choose healthy foods, your food plan, together with regular physical activity, helps you:

- Keep glucose levels in target
- Maintain healthy levels of cholesterol and triglyceride
- Reach or maintain a healthy weight
- Prevent or delay diabetes complications

Carbohydrate Foods and Glucose

Food contains carbohydrate, protein, and fat. Carbohydrate foods (carbs) affect glucose levels the most. Carbs are digested and changed into glucose. If the body doesn't use glucose properly, glucose stays in the bloodstream and glucose levels get too high.

Carbs provide energy and contain important nutrients, fiber, vitamins, and minerals. They are good for you and should be included at every meal.

Carbs include:

- Bread, tortillas, crackers, and flat breads

- Rice, pasta, and cereal

- Corn, potatoes, peas, and red and black beans

- Fruits and juices

- Milk and yogurt

- Candy, cookies, ice cream, and other desserts

- Soft drinks (not diet), sports drinks, lemonade, and sweetened tea

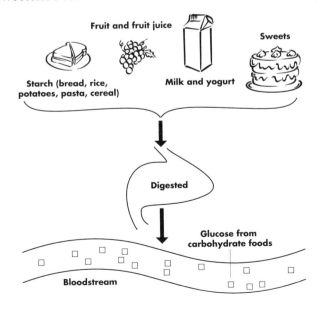

Foods with Little or No Carb

Meats, poultry, fish, and fats do not contain carb and therefore have little effect on your glucose level. Still, they are an important part of your food plan because they provide protein and other nutrients. Choose lean meats and healthy fats to help protect your heart.

Most vegetables have very little carb in them, so they do not affect your glucose level. Vegetables, such as salad greens, broccoli, carrots, and peppers, come packed with vitamins, minerals, and fiber. They are great additions to meals and snacks; eat as many as you like.

How Carb Counting Works

Carb counting is a way for you to keep track of how much carbohydrate you eat at meals and snacks. You will be given a list of foods that contain carbohydrate.

If you eat too many carbs at one time, your glucose level may go too high. The illustrations below show two examples of carbs at lunch.

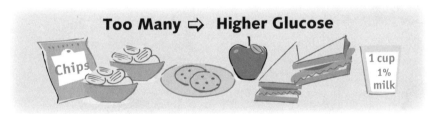

It's best to eat smaller amounts of carbs spread out over at least three meals. This helps you keep your glucose level in target.

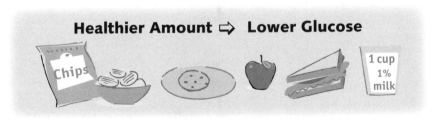

If you don't eat enough carbs and you are taking certain diabetes medications, your glucose level may go too low.

What Is a Carb Choice?

You can count carbs by grams or choices. One "carb choice" is a serving of food or drink that has about 15 grams of carb. Your food plan tells you how much carb to have at each meal or snack. You decide which foods you want to eat.

1 carbohydrate choice =

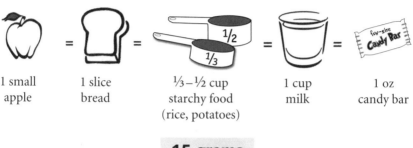

| 1 small apple | 1 slice bread | ⅓–½ cup starchy food (rice, potatoes) | 1 cup milk | 1 oz candy bar |

15 grams

Now that you know what a carb choice is, the next step is to learn how to count carbs. See the examples below.

- One small apple equals 1 carb choice or 15 grams of carb.

- Two small apples equal 2 carb choices or 30 grams of carb.

- One large apple equals 2 carb choices or 30 grams of carb.

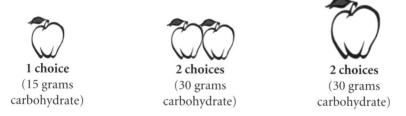

| 1 choice (15 grams carbohydrate) | 2 choices (30 grams carbohydrate) | 2 choices (30 grams carbohydrate) |

Each time you eat, add up your carbs. Eating the amount that matches your food plan helps you keep your glucose level in target.

Both of the meals below contain about the same amount of carb. While the foods are different, each meal counts as 4 carb choices or about 60 grams of carb.

Lunch 1	Carb Choices	Carb Grams
1 turkey sandwich (2 slices bread)	2	30
1 small apple	1	15
1 cup milk	1	12
Total Carbs	**4 choices**	**57 grams**

Lunch 2	Carb Choices	Carb Grams
2 cups soup	2	30
6 soda crackers	1	15
Green salad with dressing	0	0
½ cup low-fat ice cream	1	15
Total Carbs	**4 choices**	**60 grams**

Practice Carb Counting

How many choices or grams are included in each sample meal? You may use *My Food Plan* or another list of carb foods to help you.

Breakfast	Amount	Carb Amount Choices or Grams
Orange juice	½ cup	_____
Cereal, cooked	1 cup	_____
Milk, skim	1 cup	_____
Wheat toast	1 slice	_____
Peanut butter	2 tsp	_____
Banana	1 medium	
	Total Carbs =	_____
Lunch or Evening Meal	**Amount**	**Carb Amount**
Roast beef	3 oz	_____
Baked potato	1 medium (6 oz)	_____
Green beans, cooked	½ cup	_____
Lettuce salad	small	_____
w/Italian dressing	2 Tbsp	_____
Dinner roll	1 small (1 oz)	_____
Butter	1 tsp	_____
Cookies, small	2	_____
Coffee	1 cup	_____
	Total Carbs =	_____
Snack	**Amount**	**Carb Amount**
Popcorn, microwave	½ bag	_____
	Total Carbs =	_____

Can you figure out the total carb choices or grams for this fast-food meal, using the information you have?

Fast-Food Meal	Amount	Carb Amount
Cheeseburger	1	_____
French fries	medium	_____
Diet soft drink	16 oz	_____
Reduced-fat ice cream cone	small	_____
	Total Carbs =	_____

Do these meals fit into your plan? See page 106 in the *Appendix* for answers.

Understanding Food Labels

Food labels have the information you need for counting carbs. Look for the section labeled *Nutrition Facts*. To count carbs, you need to know:

- Serving size

- Servings per package

- Total carbohydrate (listed in grams for one serving)

Look at the label on the next page, and then take the "Food Label Quiz" below. If you choose to count carb choices, use the following chart to convert carb grams to carb choices. Some people prefer to count carb grams. Use the method that is easiest for you.

Carb Grams		Carb Choices
0–5	=	0 choices
6–10	=	½ choice
11–20	=	1 choice
21–25	=	1½ choices
26–35	=	2 choices
36–40	=	2½ choices
41–50	=	3 choices
51–55	=	3½ choices
56–65	=	4 choices
66–70	=	4½ choices
71–80	=	5 choices

Food Label Quiz:

1. What is the serving size? _____

2. How many servings are in each package? _____

3. How many grams of carb does one serving contain? _____

4. One serving is _____ carb choices.

Look for answers on page 106 in the *Appendix*.

Serving Size

All the information on the label is for this portion. If you eat double the serving size, you will double the carbs. You will also double the calories and other nutrients.

Servings Per Package

The number of servings contained in the package.

Total Carbohydrate

The total grams of carb found in one serving. The dietary fiber and sugar are included in this total, so don't count them twice.

Dietary Fiber

Fiber is included in "Total Carbohydrate," but does not affect glucose levels. If your food serving has five or more grams of fiber, subtract half the grams of fiber from the total grams of carb.

Nutrition Facts

Serving Size 1 bar (36g)
Servings Per Package 6

Amount Per Serving

Calories 140 Calories from Fat 25

	%Daily Value*
Total Fat 3g	5%
Saturated Fat 0.5g	3%
Cholesterol 5mg	2%
Sodium 110mg	5%
Total Carbohydrate 27g	9%
Dietary Fiber 2g	4%
Sugars 9g	
Protein 2g	16%

Vitamin A 15%	•	Vitamin C 0%	
Calcium 20%	•	Iron 10%	

* Percent daily values are based on a 2,000 calorie diet. Your daily values may be higher or lower depending on your calorie needs:

	Calories:	2,000	2,500
Total Fat	Less than	65g	80g
Sat Fat	Less than	20g	25g
Cholesterol	Less than	300mg	300mg
Sodium	Less than	2400mg	2400mg
Total Carbohydrate		300g	375g
Dietary Fiber		25g	30g

Calories per gram:
Fat 9 • Carbohydrate 4 • Protein 4

Your Personal Food Plan

A dietitian will design a food plan specifically for you. It may change over time.

The table below gives general guidelines for how much carb to include at meals. Food plans on average include 3 to 4 carb choices (45 to 60 grams) at each meal. You may need more or less, depending on your personal goals and health needs. A food plan will include at least 2 carb choices (30 grams) at each meal for good nutrition.

General Carb Guidelines for Each Meal

	To Lose Weight	To Maintain Weight	For the Very Active
Women	2–3 choices (30–45 grams)	3–4 choices (45–60 grams)	4–5 choices (60–75 grams)
Men	3–4 choices (45–60 grams)	4–5 choices (60–75 grams)	4–6 choices (60–90 grams)

Spread out your meals and snacks. This will help you manage your glucose levels. Try to eat main meals at least four hours apart. Wait at least two hours after a meal, if you choose to eat a snack.

Snacking

Snacks are not required just because you have diabetes. However, many people choose to eat them because they:

- Like them

- Are hungry between meals

- Want to avoid overeating at meals

- Are more active than usual

- Have low glucose between meals

Snacks often add extra calories and fat. To avoid gaining weight, keep portions small (1 to 2 carb choices or 15 to 30 grams) and choose low-fat foods.

See a list of healthy snacks in the *Appendix* on pages 113–114. Low-carb or no-carb options are included, but these are often higher in fat and calories.

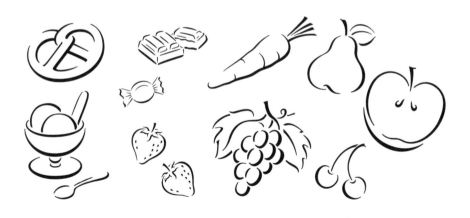

Keeping a Food Record

It's a good idea to keep a food record when you are first following your food plan or when you think your treatment plan might need changing. Keeping a record of what, when, how much you eat, and your activity level will help you and your dietitian design or change your food plan. You may also want to make notes about your feelings and experiences during this time.

Together, accurate food, activity, and glucose records provide important information. They help you see what is working for you and what isn't.

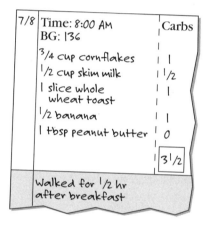

7/8	Time: 8:00 AM BG: 136	Carbs
	3/4 cup cornflakes	1
	1/2 cup skim milk	1/2
	1 slice whole wheat toast	1
	1/2 banana	1
	1 tbsp peanut butter	0
		3 1/2
	Walked for 1/2 hr after breakfast	

The Benefits of Physical Activity

It's hard to imagine anything better for you than physical activity. This doesn't change when you have diabetes. Food provides energy to your body while physical activity uses that energy.

Even a small increase in physical activity can have a big effect on your diabetes and your health. It can:

- Lower your glucose levels

- Help your body use insulin better

- Create a feeling of health and well-being

- Increase your energy

- Improve your heart health and lower blood pressure

- Increase your strength, endurance, and flexibility

- Help with weight loss or weight maintenance

Physical activity doesn't have to be hard to be good. Anything that gets you moving is a positive step.

"The Activity Pyramid" on the next page shows many ways to include activity in your life. Circle any that you like to do. Or write in your own! The best activity is the one you will do.

Your glucose may go too low during or after activity if you take certain kinds of diabetes pills or insulin. Carry a small carb snack (1 carb choice or 15 grams) with you when you exercise in case this happens.

Physical activity is any movement of your body that uses energy. Housecleaning, mowing the grass, or walking at the mall all count. Current guidelines* recommend at least 30 minutes of activity most days of the week. It can be one 30-minute session or three 10-minute sessions.

If you haven't exercised in a while and are ready to start, check with your provider. If you are just getting started, begin with 10 or 15 minutes and gradually increase as you are able.

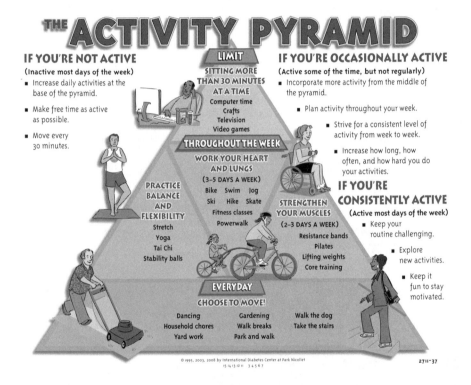

THE ACTIVITY PYRAMID

IF YOU'RE NOT ACTIVE
(Inactive most days of the week)
- Increase daily activities at the base of the pyramid.
- Make free time as active as possible.
- Move every 30 minutes.

LIMIT
SITTING MORE THAN 30 MINUTES AT A TIME
Computer time
Crafts
Television
Video games

THROUGHOUT THE WEEK
WORK YOUR HEART AND LUNGS
(3-5 DAYS A WEEK)
Bike   Swim   Jog
Ski   Hike   Skate
Fitness classes
Powerwalk

PRACTICE BALANCE AND FLEXIBILITY
Stretch
Yoga
Tai Chi
Stability balls

STRENGTHEN YOUR MUSCLES
(2-3 DAYS A WEEK)
Resistance bands
Pilates
Lifting weights
Core training

EVERYDAY
CHOOSE TO MOVE!
Dancing   Gardening   Walk the dog
Household chores   Walk breaks   Take the stairs
Yard work   Park and walk

IF YOU'RE OCCASIONALLY ACTIVE
(Active some of the time, but not regularly)
- Incorporate more activity from the middle of the pyramid.
- Plan activity throughout your week.
- Strive for a consistent level of activity from week to week.
- Increase how long, how often, and how hard you do your activities.

IF YOU'RE CONSISTENTLY ACTIVE
(Active most days of the week)
- Keep your routine challenging.
- Explore new activities.
- Keep it fun to stay motivated.

© 1995, 2003, 2008 by International Diabetes Center at Park Nicollet
15 14 13 12 11   3 4 5 6 7   2711-37

---

* Guidelines developed in 2005 by the U.S. Department of Health and Human Services and the U.S. Department of Agriculture

Planning for Success

By now you know that taking care of your diabetes means making some changes. You will develop new behaviors, such as counting carbs and testing your glucose. It also may be time to change some old habits.

Change is challenging for most people, especially when we change or develop a new behavior. We usually need time and effort to adjust.

Thought and planning can help you meet the challenge of change. It can help you:

- Decide what you are going to do and how

- Identify and plan for things that might get in the way

- Recognize when you need help and support

- Appreciate your success

Between now and *Session 2*, consider the questions on the following page. (Write whatever you want. No one else will see it.)

The information you collect will help you create a plan for success at the next session.

As I look at making changes:

1. What old habits might be difficult for me to change?

2. What new behaviors would I like to start?

3. What might get in my way of making these changes?

4. What or who might support me?

5. Use this space to write down some of your thoughts and feelings about living with diabetes.

Until We Meet Again

Please bring the following to your next appointment:

- This book

- Your food and activity record

- Your diabetes record book

- Your glucose meter, test strips, and control solution

- Your spouse or friend (optional)

- Your questions

- Other: _____

What to do between now and your next visit:

☐ Test your glucose level every day at the recommended testing times.

☐ Record your glucose readings in your diabetes record book.

☐ Complete your food and activity record for at least three days.

☐ Stay active or become more active.

☐ Think about the new behaviors you have recently started and what else you might want to work on.

☐ Make notes about challenges to taking care of your diabetes.

☐ Other: _____

Welcome

In this session, you will:

- Evaluate your glucose test results

- Learn how to care for your glucose meter and test strips

- Learn the causes, symptoms, and treatment for low and high glucose

- Learn how illness and stress affect glucose levels

- Discover tips for eating anywhere with confidence

- Learn how alcohol affects your glucose

- Discover how regular physical activity helps glucose levels

- Gain confidence in your ability to deal with your diabetes

- Create a diabetes success plan

BASICS Checklist

Be sure to ask your care team any questions you have about:

☐ Meters, glucose testing, or targets

☐ Diabetes medications

☐ Carb foods, carb counting, or reading food labels

☐ Physical activity

Reviewing Your Diabetes Record Book

Your glucose test numbers show how well your diabetes treatment plan is working.

The goal is to have at least half (50%) of your glucose tests in target at each of the times you test.

Example:
Over the last 2 weeks:

Tests in Target		Total Number of Tests		Tests in Target (%)
20	÷	40	=	0.50
				(which means 50% are in target)

Now look at **your** tests for the last one to two weeks. Complete the following steps.

1. Highlight and count all the tests in the target range.

2. Count the total number of tests you recorded.

3. Divide the number of tests in target by the total number of tests.

Fill in the blank spaces in the chart below.

My Results:
Over the last 2 weeks:

Tests in Target		Total Number of Tests		Tests in Target (%)
_____	÷	_____	=	_____

Were at least 50% of your glucose readings in target?

☐ No, the result is less than 50% (0.5). I need to continue to test *three times a day*, every day.

☐ Yes, the result is 50% (0.5) or higher. I can test less often: *three times a day*, two or three days a week.

Achieving Accurate Results

You and your care team use your testing results to make decisions about your treatment. For this reason, it's important that your test results are accurate.

Your meter needs maintenance to continue working properly. Keep it clean and check it using control solution. Directions for doing this come with your meter.

How do you know if your meter is working?

- Match the code number on your meter to your test strips, if needed.

- Use the control solution when you:

  ▷ Open a new container of test strips

  ▷ Get a result that doesn't seem right to you

  ▷ Accidentally drop your meter

If you have questions about your meter, call the toll-free number on the back of it. Meter companies have assistance available 24 hours a day.

How do you know your test strips are OK to use?

- Keep strips covered, dry, and in original packaging until you use them.

- Check the package instructions for how long to keep strips after you open the package. Write the date on the container so that you know when to start using new strips.

- Do not use strips after the expiration date.

Low Glucose

Your glucose level goes up and down throughout the day. That's normal. It goes up when you eat and down as your body uses glucose for energy.

If you take certain kinds of diabetes pills or insulin, your glucose can drop too low. Low glucose is called *hypoglycemia.*

For most people with diabetes, a glucose level below 70 mg/dL is too low. Your care team might give you a different number based on your health needs. You can work to prevent low glucose levels once you know what causes them. If you are not taking diabetes medication, you probably won't be at risk for low glucose.

Possible Causes of Low Glucose

LOW

Blood Glucose

- Eating less carbohydrate than usual

- Skipping or delaying a meal or snack

- Being more active than usual

- Taking too much diabetes medication

Symptoms of Low Glucose

If your glucose is low, you may feel:

| Weak, shaky, or lightheaded | Sweaty or clammy | Irritated | Confused | Hungry |

You may experience other symptoms, including a racing heartbeat or numb or tingling lips.

Treating Low Glucose

Whenever you feel symptoms, test your glucose right away. If it is below 70 mg/dL, eat or drink a carb choice (15 grams) to bring your glucose back up. Your care team may give you a different number than 70 mg/dL for treating lows.

Routine 15 to Treat Lows

- When you feel low symptoms, do a glucose test.

- If your glucose is low, eat or drink 15 grams of carb.

- Wait 15 minutes and do another test.

- If your glucose is still low, eat or drink another 15 grams of carb.

- Wait 15 minutes. Test again. If necessary, eat or drink another 15 grams of carb.

- If your glucose level remains low after three treatments, call your provider or 911.

Good Choices for Treating Lows

Each of the following choices has 15 grams of carb (1 carb choice):

- ½ cup fruit juice

- 1 cup milk

- ½ cup regular soft drink (not diet)

- 3 or 4 glucose tablets

- 2 or 3 hard candies

If you can't test and you think that your glucose is low, treat the symptoms. Low glucose can be dangerous if not treated. Always carry a carb source with you!

High Glucose

Your treatment plan is aimed at keeping your glucose in target. Even so, it will sometimes be high. This is called *hyperglycemia.*

Possible Causes of High Glucose

- Eating more carbohydrate than usual

- Being less active than usual

- Emotional stress or physical stress, such as illness or recent surgery

- Forgetting to take diabetes medication

- Not taking enough diabetes medication

HIGH

Blood
Glucose

Symptoms of High Glucose

Usually glucose has to be very high for symptoms to appear. While not everyone has symptoms with high glucose, those who do may:

- Feel thirsty

- Feel tired

- Go to the bathroom more often than usual

- Have blurry vision

When you are not sick, physical activity is a good way to bring high glucose back down. If your glucose is too high too often, your treatment plan needs to change. This may involve changes to your food plan, activity level, or your diabetes medication. You and your care team will decide what changes to make.

High Glucose and Stress

Stress can lead to high glucose. It can also interfere with taking care of your diabetes. Then, it is even harder to keep your glucose levels in target. And that causes more stress!

Both negative and positive events can cause stress. Dealing with a loved one's illness or death, moving to a new home, starting a new job, raising children, and reaching retirement age may all be stressful.

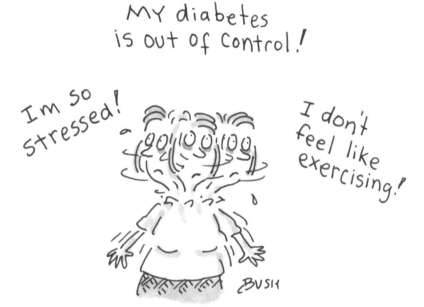

Try to find ways to keep your life balanced. Spend more time doing things you enjoy. Find time to relax.

Stress is a natural part of life. It's how you manage it that matters.

When You Are Sick

Pay special attention to your diabetes when you have the flu, a cold, or an infection. Any illness puts added stress on your body and can raise glucose levels. Glucose levels can get high very fast, so testing is important. To keep track of it, you will need to check your glucose more than usual during this time.

Follow your food plan, if you can. If your stomach is upset, it's still important to eat or drink small amounts of carb food. Your body needs fuel to help with healing. See the list below for some good options.

Carb Choices for Sick Days

Each of the following food or beverage choices has 15 grams of carb (1 carb choice):

- ½ cup regular soft drink
- 6 saltine crackers
- 1 slice toast
- 1 cup soup with noodles or rice
- ½ cup sweetened gelatin
- 1 Popsicle (single, not sugar-free)
- ½ cup ice cream or frozen yogurt
- 1 Tbsp honey or sugar
- ¼ cup sherbet

Here are some guidelines to follow when you are sick:

- If you take a diabetes medication, continue the usual dose. Your provider will tell you if it needs to be changed.

- Check and record your glucose level every four hours.

- Drink plenty of sugar-free, caffeine-free liquids to replace body fluids lost during illness. Examples include water, broth, and tea.

Call your provider if:

- Most of your glucose results are over 250 mg/dL for more than two days in a row

- Your glucose falls below 70 mg/dL more than once during your illness, and you have symptoms of hypoglycemia (low glucose)

- You are vomiting or have persistent diarrhea

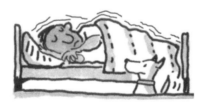

Your Diabetes Success Plan

A success plan is a tool to help you make changes to live better with diabetes. It helps you focus on your successes. When you focus on what you are doing well, it helps keep you motivated.

A success plan is practical. It is something you think you can really do. Look at the following "practical" plan. How is it different from the "not practical" plan?

Practical plan	Not practical plan
An inactive person writes, "I will walk for at least 15 minutes three days each week for the next three months."	An inactive person writes, "I will jog three miles five days a week."

A useful plan is measurable. It gives you a way to recognize your success.

Measurable plan	Not measurable plan
"I will limit my snacks to one or two carb choices."	"I will eat better snacks from now on."

Your success plan states what you will do and when you will do it. Think about your health needs, schedule, resources, support, and what you are able to do. Think about what *you* want, instead of what others want you to do. What will help you feel good and achieve your goal?

If your plan is practical and fits into your life, you will be more successful.

Many people think their plan *should* be this or *should* be that. This is *your* plan. You decide what you need to do for yourself. Based on what you've learned so far in these classes, what would you like to work on or change? Pick something that you really want to do and will feel good about doing.

To help you decide on a plan, review your answers on page 34. Also, check your diabetes record book for any notes you made.

Once you select a plan, ask yourself:

How *important* is it to me to make this change?

0........1........2........3........4........5........6........7........8........9......10
Not at all   Very

If you answered 5 or less, you may not be ready to take on this plan right now for many reasons. It may not be the right time. You may feel pressure to do what someone else wants you to do. This suggests that a different plan might be more important to you right now.

If you answered 6 or more, it looks like your plan is important to you, so go onto the next question.

How *confident* am I that I can make this change?

0........1........2........3........4........5........6........7........8........9......10
Not at all   Very

If you answered 5 or less, is there something you could do to feel more confident? Would more information help? Would it help to talk with someone who has done this successfully or someone on your care team? Once you explore support options, rate your confidence level again. If you still are not feeling confident, consider choosing another plan.

If it is important to you and you are confident that you can do it, it is much more likely that you will!

Getting the Most Out of Your Food Plan

Most people have a mixture of successes and challenges when following a food plan. Some changes come easily. Others are more challenging. It's a balance that you might have to work on every day.

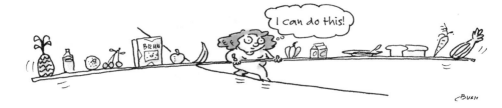

Carb counting is important to food planning success. Other good skills are:

- Making healthy food choices

- Estimating portions

- Dining out successfully

Once you learn these skills, you can eat anywhere with confidence. They will help you follow your food plan in any situation.

Making Healthy Food Choices

Good nutrition is important for everyone, whether or not they have diabetes. Eating a variety of nutritious foods helps you feel good and stay healthy.

Even though we know how to make good food choices, sometimes we don't do it. When we get busy, we might have to make quick meal decisions. Rather than make a run for fast food, it may help to plan meals or snacks ahead of time.

Healthy food choices start with fresh vegetables and fruits. They are high in vitamins, minerals, and fiber, and are low in sodium (salt). They add variety, color, and flavor to meals and make good low-fat, low-calorie snacks.

Eating at least three servings of whole grains daily—wheat, oats, barley, or rye—is good for overall health. Choose from a variety of whole-grain breads, cereals, crackers, brown rice, or whole-wheat pasta. Look for the words *whole grain* on the label.

Milk, yogurt, and other dairy products are great sources of calcium. Consider including them in your food plan each day. If it's hard to fit milk into your food plan at meals, have it as a snack instead.

Choose fresh, unprocessed foods whenever possible. Choosing low-fat foods is good for your heart, as well as for your diabetes. You'll learn more about eating for heart health in *Session 3*.

Estimating Portions

Estimating food portions can be tricky. It's best to practice for a while to develop this skill. Try this at home:

- Measure ⅓ cup of cooked pasta and put it on a dinner plate. Now measure out 1 cup of cooked pasta. Can you see the difference? One-third cup is 1 carb choice (15 grams) while 1 cup is 3 carb choices (45 grams).

- Measure a 2-inch long potato. This is 1 carb choice (15 grams). If you eat a 4-inch long potato, it's 2 carb choices (30 grams).

Remember to regularly check the accuracy of your measuring and estimating skills. Portions tend to grow over time!

The "Helping Hands" method below is another way to estimate portions.

Note: Everyone's hand is a different size, so start by measuring the amounts (see graphic to the right) and compare them to your hand. If needed, make adjustments to match your hand.

Helping Hands

½ cup is about the size and thickness of your palm without the fingers (examples: peas, corn)

1 cup is about the size of your fist (examples: milk, soup, squash)

1 snack choice is a moderate handful (examples: chips, pretzels)

1 bread choice is about the size of your open palm and half your fingers (examples: bread slice, tortilla, pancake, waffle)

1 tablespoon is about the size of your thumb (examples: jelly, syrup, honey)

Dining Out Successfully

You can enjoy eating away from home and still have good glucose control. The challenge is to eat the amount of carb listed in your food plan.

Restaurant portions often are large and high in fat and calories. See "Dining Out Favorites" on pages 115–116 in the *Appendix*. If you eat out often, consider buying a reference book that has the carb and fat content of your favorite restaurant meals. You can also find nutrition information for specific chain restaurants on the Internet.

Use the following guidelines to make your dining out experience a better one.

Choose low-fat. Select broiled, baked, grilled, or steamed menu items. Remove the skin from poultry and trim off visible fat from meat. Select a baked potato instead of au gratin. Use one pat of butter or margarine instead of two or three. If you choose a higher-fat item, eat less fat at other meals that day.

Pay attention to portions. Consider splitting a meal; ask for a half portion or have your server place half of your meal in a takeout container before you even begin eating. Avoid "super" or "deluxe" menu items. Choose wisely at buffets. Ask the server if you are unsure about portion sizes. Remember, you can't "save" carb choices from one meal and have them at another.

Ask for what you want. Restaurants want you to enjoy your meal, so, don't be afraid to ask for substitutions. Try a salad or fruit instead of French fries. Have salad dressing or toppings on the side. You'll probably use less if you add it yourself.

Enjoy yourself. If you sometimes eat too much, it's OK! A little extra activity may help. If you often overeat, think about why, and then plan ahead. For example, if you usually overeat when having pizza, enjoy a salad first.

If you frequently eat out and have difficulty choosing healthy foods or portions, consider eating out less. Plan ahead. Pack your lunch or carry a snack. This may help lessen the temptation to indulge in high-carb, high-fat foods in the break room, vending machines, or restaurants.

To make healthier food choices, look for hints in menu descriptions. Restaurant foods can stump even those with the best carb counting skills. For example, many Asian dishes or barbeque sauces are thickened or sweetened with carbohydrate. Meal sized salads may contain many carbohydrate ingredients that tend to add up quickly. These include: croutons, tortilla strips, beans, and sweetened dressings.

Choosing menu items that are not too high in fat or calories can be difficult. The best clues are often in the description of the menu items.

Choose More	Choose Less
Blackened	Au gratin/scalloped
Grilled, baked, or broiled	Breaded
Poached	Buttered or buttery
Sautéed	Cream or cheese sauce
Steamed	Deep fried or French fried
	Gravy or hollandaise
	Rich or smothered

The following four meals are between 3–5 carb choices (45–75 grams). Portions served at restaurants may be larger than this. Use this as a guide to help you dine out more successfully.

Salad Meal	Carb Choices	Carb Grams
Large chicken caesar salad with dressing/croutons	2	30
Small dinner roll	1	15
½ cup mixed fruit	1	15
Iced tea	0	0
	4	60

Asian Meal	Carb Choices	Carb Grams
1½ cups chicken stir fry	1½	23
⅔ cup fried rice	2	30
1 egg roll	1½	23
Ice water with lemon	0	0
	5	76

Meat Meal	Carb Choices	Carb Grams
Sirloin steak	0	0
½ large baked potato	2	30
1 bread stick	1	15
5 oz wine	0	0
	3	45

Italian Meal	Carb Choices	Carb Grams
1 cup pasta	3	45
½ cup red sauce	1	15
Meatballs	0	0
Dinner salad with Italian dressing	0	0
1 slice Italian bread	1	15
	5	75

Diabetes and Alcohol

Dining out and alcohol often go together. If you drink alcohol, take time to understand how it affects your diabetes and health.

Alcohol does not change into glucose, but it does prevent your body from making glucose. When you're drinking alcohol, glucose can go too low, especially if you haven't eaten.

Alcohol may also raise your blood fat levels (triglycerides). Each drink contains 100 to 200 calories.

Guidelines for Safe Alcohol Use

- Drink alcohol only when your diabetes is under control.

- Drink alcohol with carb foods, not on an empty stomach.

- Limit the amount to one serving (women) or two servings (men).

- Be alert to symptoms of low glucose. Monitor glucose more closely after drinking.

- Wear medical identification. Low glucose may be mistaken for intoxication.

- When taking the diabetes pill metformin, limit yourself to no more than two drinks because it poses additional health risks.

Alcohol	1 Serving	Grams of Carb
Beer, regular	12 oz	13
Beer, light	12 oz	5–11 (check label)
Liquor, hard	1½ oz	Trace
Liqueurs	½ oz	18
Wine	5 oz	Trace

Some alcoholic beverages, like regular beer, do contain carb and may raise your glucose levels. For this reason, light beer, diet soft drinks, and diet tonics are better choices.

Get Your Body Moving

Physical activity starts when you get up in the morning and continues as you go about your daily life. You already know it lowers glucose levels. *Regular* activity helps your body use insulin better. This means you are active at least three or four days each week, spread throughout the week.

One way to increase your activity level is to recognize the ways you are already active and increase the time. So, if you walk 15 minutes a day, increase to 25 or 30 minutes. Another way is to change some of the inactive things you do so they are more active. Look at the table below for ideas. Can you add any of your own ideas?

Less Activity	More Activity
Watch TV	Walk in place while watching television
Hire someone to clean	Clean your own house
Lunch with a friend or coworker	Walk with a friend or coworker at lunch time
Take the car to the carwash	Wash your own car
Wait for an appointment or flight	Take a walk while waiting
Hire someone to mow your lawn	Mow your own lawn
Work at the computer	Get up and move every 30 minutes
Read	Listen to an audio book while walking
Take the elevator	Take the stairs
Golf using a golf cart	Walk instead of using a golf cart

Working with Your Diabetes Success Plan

Think of ways to make your success plan work for you. For example, ask a friend to walk with you during lunch, check out the carb count of your favorite restaurant food, or keep your glucose meter and strips on your bedside table to remind you to test in the morning.

Commit yourself to your plan. Saying you will "try" is another way of saying you probably won't do it. Commitment helps turn something you think you might do into something you believe you will do.

After working with your food plan for at least a month, consider the questions on the following page. (Write whatever you want. No one else will see it.)

Your answers to these questions are clues to what is going well for you. Celebrate your success and make the most out of your positive experiences. You are much more likely to stay motivated if you take credit for your efforts.

As I begin making changes:

1. What did I gain working with my success plan?

2. What helped me with my plan?

3. What was my biggest challenge?

4. Do I need to adjust my plan? If so, what change will I make?

Until We Meet Again

Bring the following to your next appointment:

- This book
- Your food and activity record
- Your diabetes record book
- Your diabetes success plan
- Questions and experiences to share
- Other: _____

What to do between now and your next visit:

☐ Test your glucose level at the recommended testing times.

☐ Record your glucose readings in your diabetes record book.

☐ Complete a food and activity record on at least three of the days you test.

☐ Evaluate your diabetes success plan by answering the questions on page 57.

☐ Other: _____

Welcome

In this session, you will:

- Understand why glucose may be out of target

- Learn how diabetes changes over time

- Identify diabetes complications and learn about prevention

- Learn about blood pressure, cholesterol, and heart health

- Learn about lowering dietary fat and sodium

- Understand the benefits of physical activity for heart health

- Recognize the successes and challenges with your success plan

BASICS Checklist

Be sure to ask your care team any questions about:

☐ Your treatment plan or food

☐ Glucose testing results

☐ Sick day management

☐ Carb counting, dining out, or alcohol

☐ The effect of activity on glucose

☐ Your diabetes success plan

Success Plan Checkpoint

Living well with diabetes involves a series of successes. Each glucose test is a success. Each carb counted is a success. Each choice to walk is a success.

You chose a success plan in *Session 2*. By now you have been working with it for several months. How is it going?

You have probably learned a lot from working with your plan. Maybe some things about it have been easier for you than others.

Now is a good time to think about what you have learned. Think back over the past several weeks. Taking this time to reflect can help you to continue to work on your plan or choose a different plan.

You may have decided your plan isn't a good fit right now. Changing behaviors often means changing plans.

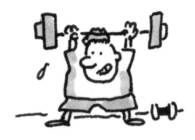

Name at least one thing you would like to celebrate.

How do you want to celebrate this success?

Recognizing your challenges is part of success, too. When you know what your challenges are, you can choose what you want to do about them. Awareness gives you strength.

Be kind to yourself as you work with your plan. Share your victories. Give yourself credit for any effort you make.

Reviewing Your Diabetes Record Book

The goal is to have at least half (50%) of your glucose tests in target at each of the times you test.

Example:
Over the last 2 weeks:

Tests in Target		Total Number of Tests		Tests in Target (%)
12	÷	16	=	0.75
				(which means 75% are in target)

Now look at your tests for the last two weeks. Complete the following steps.

1. Highlight and count all the tests in the target range.

2. Count the total number of tests you recorded.

3. Divide the number of tests in target by the total number of tests.

Fill in the blank spaces in the chart below.

My Results:
Over the last 2 weeks:

Tests in Target		Total Number of Tests		Tests in Target (%)
_____	÷	_____	=	_____

Were at least 50% of your glucose readings in target? Check one of the answers below.

❏ No, the result is less than 50% (0.5). I need to continue to test *three times a day*, every day.

❏ Yes, the result is 50% (0.5) or higher. I can test less often: *three times a day*, two or three days a week.

Using Your Glucose Numbers

Your test results can help you to understand how your glucose responds to different foods, to physical activity, and to stress.

Let's look at an example. Suppose you have a high glucose level before dinner. Several things might have caused it. Maybe you:

- Ate a big lunch that day

- Missed your usual physical activity that afternoon

- Are coming down with a cold

- Had an extra afternoon snack

- Forgot to take your diabetes medication

To determine the actual cause, it helps to remember everything you did and everything you ate. That can be hard. Your record book is a great place to keep notes about things that might affect your numbers. When a number is out of target, this can help you figure out why. Knowing why helps prevent it from happening again. See the example below.

You may learn that portions of certain foods cause glucose to go high. Or you may learn that a brisk walk brings a high level down.

Evening Meal
Food/Amount

	Time: 6 p.m. BG: 125/208	Carbs
	2 cups spaghetti with sauce	6 1
	Salad with lowfat dressing	
	1 slice of french bread	1
	iced tea	
		8

Rained—Didn't walk

Holidays, parties, vacations, restaurant meals, and illness can all disrupt usual schedules. Learning from past experience can help you deal with these occasions and prevent high glucose readings.

Low glucose readings may occur if you are taking insulin or certain diabetes pills (see page 108–110). If you have low glucose, review causes and treatment on pages 40–41. If you are frequently having lows, talk to your care team about possible changes to your treatment plan. Also, make sure you are including carbohydrate at each of your meals.

Sometimes you have a result that you can't explain. Follow these tips to make sure you are getting an accurate reading. Make sure:

- Your hands are clean and retest

- Your blood sample is big enough

- Your meter and test strips are working correctly (see page 39)

After an unusually high or low number, give extra attention to your testing for the next couple of days. You may notice this keeps happening at the same time of day. This is called a blood glucose pattern. Talk to one of your care team members about any patterns you see.

Diabetes Changes over Time

It is natural for diabetes to change over time. These changes happen at different times for different people.

Three types of changes happen over a number of years.

- The body's cells become resistant to the action of insulin.

- The pancreas first makes more insulin, then less and less.

- The signal from the digestive tract can weaken. Less insulin is released with meals.

As these changes happen, your treatment plan needs to change, too. You may need to add medication or change your dose.

Many people with type 2 diabetes need more than one medication. Most eventually need insulin injections. This does not mean your diabetes is getting worse. It simply means insulin is the best treatment to help keep your glucose in target.

How Diabetes Develops and Progresses

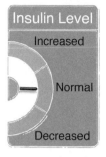

No Diabetes. The pancreas works well and makes enough insulin. The body's cells use the insulin properly. This keeps glucose levels normal.

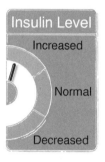

Prediabetes (10–20 years before diabetes starts). The body develops a resistance to insulin. The pancreas works harder to make more insulin. Glucose levels may go above normal but do not go high enough to become diabetes. Physical activity, healthy eating, and weight loss may help prevent or delay the start of diabetes.

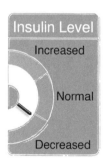

Type 2 Diabetes. The body is still resistant to insulin's effect and the pancreas can't make enough insulin. After eating, the digestive tract's signal to the pancreas can weaken and less insulin is released. Glucose goes higher. Though diabetes can be detected by blood tests at this point, it often isn't diagnosed for several years. Over time, the pancreas makes even less insulin. A combination of medication is usually needed.

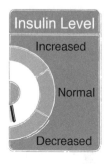

Type 2 Diabetes (progressing). The pancreas eventually may make very little insulin. When insulin production drops too low, diabetes pills alone aren't enough. At this point, insulin injections are needed. Diabetes pills that treat insulin resistance may still be needed.

Staying Healthy for a Lifetime

Because diabetes changes over time, your health care needs change too. Visit your provider every three to six months. Together, you will review your A1C and other laboratory test results. You will discuss your treatment plan and decide on any changes that may be necessary.

The "Diabetes Care Schedule for Adults" on page 112 shows the tests and exams you need to have regularly.

Complications occur when glucose levels are elevated over time. This causes damage to nerves and blood vessels. High blood pressure and abnormal cholesterol levels add to your risk. If you have concerns, talk to your provider. Treatment is available.

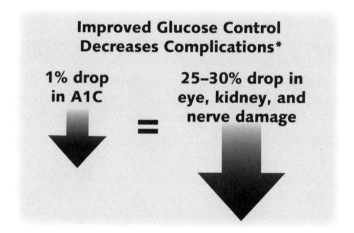

Improved Glucose Control Decreases Complications*

1% drop in A1C = **25–30% drop in eye, kidney, and nerve damage**

* Based on data from the 10-year Diabetes Control and Complications Trial, concluded in 1993, and the United Kingdom Prospective Diabetes Study, which ended in 1999.

Heart and blood vessels. Damage to the large blood vessels can lead to atherosclerosis, heart attack, and stroke.

Eyes. Damage to the small blood vessels in the eye can lead to vision problems. High blood pressure worsens eye disease.

Kidneys. Damage to the small blood vessels in the kidneys makes it hard for them to remove waste from the blood. It can also cause high blood pressure or make it worse.

Feet. Damage to the large and small blood vessels slows circulation and damages nerves in the legs and feet. This causes decreased sensation and can lead to infections that are difficult to heal.

Nerves. In addition to foot problems, nerve damage can cause difficulty with emptying the bladder and problems with digesting food properly.

Sexual function. Nerve damage can interfere with the body's sexual response and function. This can happen in both men and women.

Stomach or bowels. Nerve damage affects the digestive tract, causing food to stay in the stomach longer than normal. This leads to nausea and vomiting.

Teeth and gums. High glucose causes the natural bacteria in the mouth to multiply. This increases the risk for gum disease.

Planning for Pregnancy

Women with diabetes can get pregnant and give birth to healthy babies just as other women do. At least three months before becoming pregnant, it's important to have good glucose control. This helps achieve a successful pregnancy. Let your care team know if you are considering getting pregnant.

Healthy Feet

Healthy feet are a good reason to keep your glucose, blood pressure, and cholesterol in target. Poor circulation and nerve damage usually affect the feet and lower legs first.

Foot problems start with numbness, tingling, or pain. There may be sores that won't heal. These problems can become very serious. Taking care of your feet daily helps to prevent this.

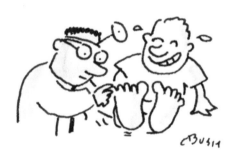

Five Steps to Good Foot Care

1. **Clean.**
   - Wash feet daily with mild soap and warm water.
   - Do not soak feet.
   - Dry feet well, especially between the toes.
   - Trim nails straight across.

2. **Check daily.**
   - Use a mirror to check hidden areas of your feet or ask for help.
   - Check inside your shoes, and shake them out to make sure there are no pebbles.

3. **Protect.**
   - Avoid temperature extremes.
   - Don't go barefoot. Wear cotton socks and shoes made of natural materials like leather.
   - Because feet swell during the day, buy shoes later in the day for a better fit.

4. **Treat.**
   - Use cream or lotion on dry feet, except between your toes.
   - Do not use chemical treatments, sharp instruments, or abrasive materials on trouble spots.
   - Clean and treat minor blisters and cuts. Watch to make sure they are healing.

5. **See your provider.**
   - Remove your shoes and socks at every visit.
   - If you have foot problems, ask your provider for a referral to a podiatrist (foot doctor).

Healthy Heart

Heart health is important because diabetes increases your risk for heart disease. Everything you do to control your glucose level helps keep your heart healthy. Other risk factors include high blood pressure, high cholesterol, and smoking. The more risk factors you have, the higher your risk for heart disease. See the chart below.

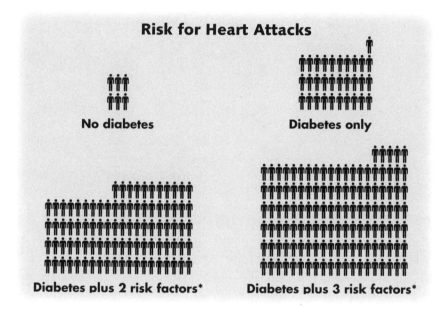

* This graphic shows the risks of heart attacks per 1,000 people over a ten-year period.

Assess Your Heart Disease Risk

Are any of the following statements true for you?

Yes : No

☐ : ☐   My A1C is 7.0% or higher.

☐ : ☐   My LDL cholesterol is 100 or higher.

☐ : ☐   My HDL cholesterol is 40 or lower.

☐ : ☐   My triglycerides are 150 or higher.

☐ : ☐   My blood pressure is 130/80 or higher.

☐ : ☐   I smoke.

☐ : ☐   I eat foods high in fat and high in saturated fat daily.

☐ : ☐   I eat less than five servings of fruits and vegetables a day.

☐ : ☐   I am not physically active on most days of the week.

☐ : ☐   One or more of my parents, brothers, or sisters has had a heart attack.

☐ : ☐   I have had a heart attack.

☐ : ☐   I have had a heart attack and have not discussed heart medications, including ACE inhibitors and beta blockers, with my doctor.

☐ : ☐   I am past menopause (women only).

Any "yes" answers are linked to an increased risk for heart disease. Talk to your provider about your risk.

Some risk factors for heart disease cannot be changed, such as your family history. Others are related to lifestyle and can be changed. Once you understand your risk factors, you can take steps to reduce them. See the following for tips on protecting your heart.

Tips for Protecting Your Heart

- Don't smoke.

- Choose low-fat foods and use low-fat cooking methods.

- Avoid foods with saturated and *trans* fats.

- Eat fewer salty foods and avoid using a salt shaker.

- Include plenty of fruits, vegetables, whole grains, and low-fat dairy products.

- Be more active.

- Lose weight (if you need to) and avoid gaining weight.

- Balance the stress in your life.

- Limit the alcohol you drink.

- Ask your provider if taking an aspirin daily would help protect your heart.

Blood Pressure and Heart Health

High blood pressure puts extra strain on the heart. It also can damage small blood vessels in the eyes and kidneys.

Blood pressure is recorded as two numbers. The upper number is the systolic blood pressure—the pressure when your heart is contracting. The lower number is the diastolic pressure—the pressure when your heart is relaxed. If either number is high, your risk for heart disease is increased.

Measure	Target	My Value
Blood pressure	Under 130/80	

If you have diabetes, your risk for developing high blood pressure is three times higher than the general population. If diet and exercise do not control your blood pressure, you may need to take one or more blood pressure medications.

Have regular blood pressure checks. Keep your blood pressure below 130/80, the target for people who have diabetes. This will help protect your heart and blood vessels.

How to Control Your Blood Pressure

- Check your blood pressure regularly. Use a home monitor or use one at a local pharmacy or shopping center.

- Bring your blood pressure records to your provider visit.

- Ask your provider about possible medications.

- Follow the guidelines on protecting your heart on page 73.

- See a dietitian for information on lowering sodium (salt) in your diet. Also, see the tips on page 75.

Lowering Salt (Sodium) for Heart Health

Lowering sodium in your diet can help lower your blood pressure. It also helps blood pressure medications work better.

- Use less salt at the table and in cooking.

- Add spices and herbs to bring out flavors in food.

- Select fresh foods instead of processed foods.

Choose more	Choose less
Fruit	Salty snack foods
Fresh/frozen vegetables (without sauces)	Canned vegetables and tomato/vegetable juice
Fresh meat, fish, and poultry	Lunch meats, bacon, and sausage
Homemade soup made with less salt	Canned or dried soup
Homemade meals	Frozen/packaged meals

When reading food labels, look for:

- Frozen dinners with less than 800 mg/sodium per serving

- Snack foods with less than 250 mg/sodium per serving

Overall, aim to keep total daily sodium to 2,300 mg or less per day, or about 800 mg at each meal.

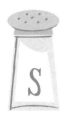

Smoking, Diabetes, and Heart Health

If you smoke, stop. One of the best things you can do for your diabetes and your heart is to not smoke. The combination of smoking and diabetes is especially dangerous. Smoking increases your risk of heart disease. It also narrows your blood vessels. This decreases blood flow to your heart and limbs, increasing your risk of complications.

Nicotine is a highly addictive drug. Yet, more than 45 million Americans have quit nicotine. Many tried to quit several times before they succeeded. A failure in the past does not mean you will fail in the future. People successfully quit smoking in different ways. Some people:

- Wean themselves off cigarettes; others quit cold turkey

- Use nicotine replacement, such as a nicotine patch, or chew nicotine gum

- Take medication prescribed by their provider

- Join programs using acupuncture or hypnosis or work with a support group

If one method doesn't work for you, don't give up. Try another method.

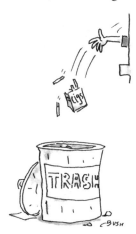

Cholesterol, Triglyceride, and Heart Health

Cholesterol and triglyceride are fatty substances called *lipids*. Your body needs them to work properly.

Your liver makes cholesterol and triglyceride. You can also get them from the foods you eat, such as meats, eggs, cheese, milk, and butter.

Small fat droplets called *lipoproteins* carry cholesterol and triglyceride in your blood. There are different types of lipoproteins.

HDL (high-density lipoprotein) is known as the *good cholesterol*. It carries cholesterol away from your body's cells. A high HDL helps keep blood vessels healthy.

- *How to increase HDL:* Be physically active, lose weight, and choose healthy fats in your diet.

LDL (low-density lipoprotein) is known as the *bad cholesterol*. It carries cholesterol and triglyceride to your body's cells. LDL cholesterol can create a waxy buildup in your blood vessels called *plaque*. A buildup of plaque is known as *atherosclerosis*. It damages your vessels and can block blood flow. A low LDL cholesterol helps protect your heart and blood vessels.

- *How to lower LDL:* Eat less saturated fat, avoid *trans* fat, lose weight, and be active regularly.

Triglyceride is fat. Your body uses it for energy and insulation. People with type 2 diabetes and insulin resistance tend to make more triglyceride. High triglyceride levels increase your risk of heart disease.

- *How to lower triglycerides:* Lose weight, eat less saturated fat, limit alcohol, and keep your glucose in target.

Have a complete cholesterol test (lipid profile) every year. The test tells you your HDL, LDL, and triglyceride values. It is usually done after fasting for at least twelve hours. Write your cholesterol levels in the chart below:

Lipid	Target (mg/dL)	My Value	Date
LDL Cholesterol	Less than 100 (with heart disease, less than 70)		
HDL Cholesterol	Greater than 40 (consider greater than 50 for women)		
Triglyceride	Less than 150		

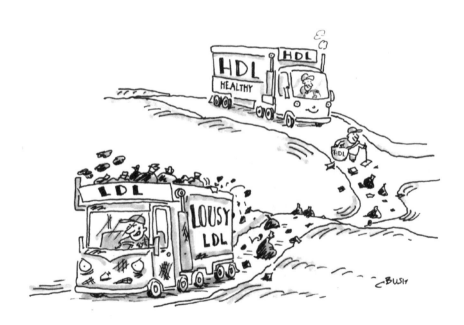

Choosing Healthy Fat

In addition to carbohydrate, fat is a source of energy for the body. Fat also provides essential fatty acids for normal body function. Fat is found in foods such as oils, snack foods, sweets, meat, and dairy products.

There are two main kinds of fat in food:

- **Unsaturated fat** lowers cholesterol. It is better for your heart and blood vessels than saturated fat. Unsaturated fat can be polyunsaturated or monounsaturated. It is usually liquid at room temperature.

- **Saturated fat** raises cholesterol. It is not good for your heart and blood vessels. It is usually solid at room temperature.

Although unsaturated fat is better for you than saturated fat, all fat is high in calories, so watch your portions.

Trans fat is another type of fat. It is a liquid fat that is made solid during food processing. *Trans* fats are very bad for your heart. They increase LDL cholesterol and decrease HDL cholesterol— just the opposite of what you want. The *Nutrition Facts* panel on the food label tells you whether a food contains *trans* fat. Partially hydrogenated oil is a common food ingredient that contains *trans* fat. Look for foods that contain zero *trans* fat.

Nutrition Facts

Serving Size 1 bar (36g)
Servings Per Package 1

Amount Per Serving

Calories 143   Calories from Fat 25

	%Daily Value*
Total Fat 3g	5%
Saturated Fat 0.5g	3%
Trans Fat 0.5g	
Cholesterol 5mg	2%
Sodium 110mg	5%
Carbohydrate 27	

Food Sources of Fat

Monounsaturated (More Healthy)	Polyunsaturated (Healthy)	Saturated (Unhealthy)	*Trans* Fat (Least Healthy)
Almonds	Corn oil	Bacon	Bakery goods
Avocados	Margarine, tub	Butter	Fried foods
Canola oil	Pumpkin seeds	Cheese	Partially hydrogenated oils
Fatty fish	Safflower oil	Coconut oil	
Olive oil	Soybean nuts	Cream	Pastries
Olives	Soybean oil	Lard	Stick margarine
Peanut butter or oil	Sunflower seeds	Meat fat	
Peanuts	Walnuts	Milk, whole or 2%	
Pecans		Palm kernel oil	
		Shortening	
		Sour cream	

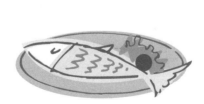

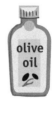

Eating Less Fat

The fat we eat can be "added" or "hidden."

Added fats are either the fat we add to food or fat that is added to the food before we buy it. Examples of fats we add include butter, dressing, or sour cream. When restaurants or food companies add fat, it is harder to see. Examples include potato chips, pastries, fried foods, or creamy pasta salads or sauces.

Hidden fats are naturally part of the foods we choose. Cheese, high-fat cuts of meat, and whole or 2% milk are examples.

Eating Less Fat for Heart Health

- Limit the fat you add to one or two servings per meal. Serving sizes are listed on your food plan. If you plan on having more fat at one meal, it is OK to save up fats from another meal.

- Cut back on foods that have fat added to them already. Watch your portions and consider using a lower fat alternative such as:

  ▷ Baked instead of fried snack chips

  ▷ Red sauce instead of cream sauce

- Limit the amount of meat or protein you eat to less than 8 ounces per day. Aim for 6 ounces or less if your cholesterol is high. Choose lean cuts of meat (round, sirloin, or tenderloin), reduced-fat cheeses, and low-fat dairy whenever possible.

The list on the next page shows heart-healthy substitutes for many high-fat foods.

High-Fat Choices	Heart-Healthy Choices
Whole or 2% milk	Skim or 1% milk
Regular cheese or cottage cheese	Part-skim cheese or low-fat cottage cheese
Regular sour cream	Light or low-fat sour cream
Butter or solid vegetable shortening	Tub margarine or cooking oil or spray
Regular salad dressing	Light or low-fat salad dressing
French fries, hash browns, or scalloped potatoes	Plain mashed or baked potato
Fried rice	Steamed or brown rice
Chicken salad sandwich or breaded chicken breast sandwich	Grilled chicken breast sandwich
Sausage, bologna, or fried chicken or fish	White turkey, chicken without skin, or broiled fish
Potato chips	Pretzels
Pasta salad made with regular mayo	Pasta salad made with low-fat mayo or olive oil

Low-Fat Cooking

- Bake, broil, or grill meats.

- Use nonstick cookware.

- Sauté food in broth or wine.

- Use cooking spray instead of oil.

- Trim fat off meat before cooking.

- Remove chicken and turkey skin, or buy skinless cuts.

Heart Healthy Quick Check

How can you make these two meals more heart healthy?

Meal 1	Amount	Heart Healthy Choice
Prime rib	10 oz	
Baked potato	6 oz (4-inches long)	
Butter	2 Tbsp	
Dinner salad	1 small	
French dressing, regular	2 Tbsp	
Dinner roll	1 roll	
Butter	2 Tbsp	
Red wine	5 oz	

Meal 2	Amount	Heart Healthy Choice
Pasta	2 cups	
Meatballs	3	
Tomato sauce	1 cup	
Soft bread stick	1 small	
Butter	1 Tbsp	
Dinner salad	1 small	
Italian dressing, regular	2 Tbsp	
Milk, 2%	1 cup	

Answers can be found on page 107 in the *Appendix*.

Stepping It Up for Heart Health

An active lifestyle can keep your heart strong. Heart healthy activity makes your heart beat faster.

Walking is one of the simplest and best physical activities for your heart. First add steps to your day and then step up the pace. Over time, try to keep up the pace for longer periods.

A pedometer is a great way to learn how active you are during a normal day. A pedometer is a small pager-like device that fits on your waistband. It counts every step you take.

You can buy pedometers at many discount or drug stores. Watching the steps add up can be very motivating. And every extra step you take is a step toward a healthier you.

Wear the pedometer for a couple of days to see how many steps you usually take. Then add steps each day. For example, if you take 2,500 steps on Monday, try to take 2,750 steps on Tuesday. One mile is about 2,000 steps.

Other physical activities that help build heart health include water aerobics, swimming, biking, and exercise videos. You can do any of these activities at a pace that's right for you and your heart.

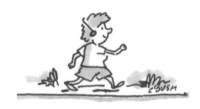

Secrets of Success

It's easy to focus on things we think we are doing wrong when working to change a behavior. We tell ourselves we're weak if we eat something fattening. We tell ourselves we're lazy if we don't exercise for a few days.

When you tell yourself that you are failing often enough, you almost surely will fail.

Instead, choose to identify what you do well. Then think of how to use your talents to support efforts to take care of yourself, such as:

- You are a *skilled* teacher or a loving parent. You notice and praise children for each small achievement. Do the same for yourself!

- You are *organized* and *efficient* at home or at work. You create simple, practical ways to get things done. Use your "can-do" attitude to fit physical activity into your day!

- You have a passion for mystery novels and usually know the ending before you get there. Use your ability to "crack the case" to help you *problem solve* your diabetes mysteries!

Answer the questions below between now and *Session 4* to explore your natural talents and gifts further.

1. What are my special skills or talents?

2. How can I use my talents to help me take care of my diabetes and to work with my success plan?

Until We Meet Again

At *Session 4*, day to day living with diabetes will be discussed. This will help you develop problem-solving skills when life doesn't go as planned. We look forward to seeing you!

Bring the following to your next appointment:

- This book

- Your diabetes record book if you have questions or concerns

- Your food & activity record if you have questions or concerns

- Your diabetes success plan

- Real-life diabetes experiences or challenges to share

- Any remaining questions you have about diabetes

What to do between now and your next visit (usually two to three months from now):

☐ Test and record your glucose.

☐ Stay active or become more active.

☐ Make heart healthy lifestyle choices.

☐ Continue to work on your diabetes success plan.

Welcome

In this session, you will:

- Develop problem-solving skills for times when glucose numbers are puzzling

- Develop strategies for creating life balance

- Learn how to identify if your treatment plan needs to change

- Develop strategies for dealing with stress, depression, and staying motivated

- Learn tips for staying active

- Build on skills for eating healthy

- Identify healthy weight-loss plans

- Gain confidence that you can succeed in caring for your diabetes

BASICS Checklist

Be sure to ask your care team any questions you have about:

☐ Your treatment plan, food plan, or success plan

☐ Your A1C or glucose testing results

☐ Blood pressure, cholesterol, smoking cessation, or foot care

☐ Heart-healthy foods

☐ The effect of physical activity on heart health

Ups and Downs of Life
with Diabetes

You've probably made a lot of changes in your life. You're testing your glucose. You may eat differently and be more active than you used to be. Maybe you take a diabetes medication now.

Most people with diabetes go through ups and downs with taking care of their diabetes. It's natural for enthusiasm and attention to fade. Life just goes on.

Like anyone striving to live a healthy lifestyle, it will help to learn how to deal with occasional drops in motivation. This is especially true when temptations and challenges surround you.

What do you do, for example, when faced with your favorite cake at a family gathering? How do you keep your treadmill from becoming an expensive coat rack?

For your health and well-being, look for ways to encourage and motivate yourself. Find people in your life who support you. Encourage them to remind you of successes. "Diabetes police" tell you what they think you are doing wrong. Hearing what you are doing *well* is more likely to motivate you.

Solving Blood Glucose Puzzles

The best thing you can do for your diabetes is to follow your treatment plan. This helps keep your glucose and A1C in target. It also helps prevent diabetes complications.

Even when you follow your treatment plan, your glucose readings can sometimes be out of target. It's easy to feel frustrated when this happens. One high reading is not a cause for alarm. Often you can explain it. If you can't, it's best just to let it go.

The best way to problem solve is to review your diabetes record book. If at least half of your readings are in target, your A1C should be in target as well. If not, you can figure out why and choose what you want to do.

If you haven't had an A1C test in the last three months, talk to your provider about having one.

You're probably already good at figuring out why your glucose gets out of target sometimes. But some numbers might still be puzzling. The following are some solutions to common problems.

One unusually high reading. This could be just a mistake. First, wash your hands and repeat the test. If it's still high, do a quality control test to make sure your meter is working right (see page 39). If everything checks out, think about what else might be going on. Review the causes of high glucose on page 42.

High readings before breakfast. A small bedtime snack doesn't usually cause morning highs. Your liver may be making extra glucose overnight. You may need a medication to help with this. You could also try adding physical activity in the evening. Getting a good night's sleep may also help.

High A1C with tests mostly in target. This usually means you have high glucose levels that you don't know about. Regular testing at different times of day can help prevent A1C surprises. Test at least three times on the days that you test—when you wake up, and then before and two hours after your main meal.

If you often have high glucose levels that you can't explain or correct, talk to your provider. You may need a change in your treatment plan.

Is Your Diabetes Treatment Plan Working?

One of the main goals of treatment is to keep your A1C from going too high. If this happens, it's time to think about changing your treatment plan.

1. What is your A1C? _____
   The chart below will help you understand *your* risk for complications.

   Find your A1C at the bottom on the chart. Draw a line up from your A1C to the line on the chart. Draw another line from that point to the risk scale on the left.

   When the A1C is 8%, as in the example below, the risk for complications is two times greater.

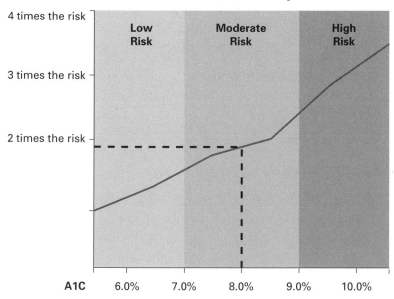

Risk for Diabetes Complications

2. What is your risk for diabetes complications?

3. Is your A1C where you want it to be?

To lower your A1C and your risk for complications, your treatment plan may need to change.

Treatment plans change because diabetes changes over time. Many people with type 2 diabetes will need two or more pills. It is also likely that they will eventually need insulin to help keep their A1C at a healthy level.

Medications don't cause complications. Not taking medications when you need them does.

Besides diabetes pills, two additional treatment options include:

1. **Injectable, Noninsulin Diabetes Medications**

These kinds of medications work like a hormone made in your body. They help people with type 2 diabetes make more insulin. Injectable, noninsulin medications include Byetta® (exenatide) and Victoza® (liraglutide). Byetta® is given twice a day. Take it one hour before morning and evening meals, but not after meals. Victoza® is given once a day at any time of day. These medications can:

- Prevent glucose from going too high after meals

- Make you feel less hungry

- Help you lose weight

- Cause nausea in some people

2. **Background (Long-Acting) Insulin**

This kind of insulin is usually taken once a day. It helps maintain a steady level of insulin in your body for about 24 hours. Background insulins include Lantus® (glargine) and Levemir® (detemir). You will still need to take diabetes pills during the day to lower your glucose after eating.

If these options don't work, your provider may recommend changing your treatment plan to include insulin at mealtimes. Check with your provider to see what will work best for you.

Managing Stress

Stress has many different causes. Because stress has a direct effect on your body, it can make glucose levels hard to control. Many people deal with stress in ways that can be harmful. They eat more because it's comforting. They exercise less to give themselves "a break." Both of these actually increase stress.

Here are a few things you can do to manage stress:

Breathe. Practice deep breathing often. Sit comfortably and breathe in slowly from your diaphragm (located right under your rib cage). Hold each breath briefly and then exhale slowly.

Sleep. Get the sleep you need; for most people this is about 7 to 8 hours. If you have trouble sleeping or regularly find yourself nodding off during the day, talk to your provider about options to help with sleep.

Laugh. Look for opportunities to laugh and have fun. Research shows that laughter lowers blood pressure and releases chemicals in your body, which can help you feel better.

Put your needs first. Ask for help when you need it. Don't be afraid to say "no." You eventually may lose the ability to help others if you are not taking care of yourself.

Relax. By relaxing, you can slow your heart and breathing rate and lower your blood pressure. Listening to music, meditating, praying, doing yoga, or reading are a few of the things that can help you relax.

Life Balance Check

Do you usually:

Yes	No	
☐	☐	Deal well with irritating life hassles?
☐	☐	Cope well with important changes in your life?
☐	☐	Feel confident in your ability to handle your personal problems?
☐	☐	Believe that things are going your way?
☐	☐	Think you are able to control irritations in your life?
☐	☐	Believe you can handle things?
☐	☐	Think you are able to control the way you spend your time?

Three or more "no" answers suggest that you have trouble coping with the stress in your life. Consider talking with your care team about options for managing stress. You can use the "Life Balance Pyramid" on the next page to help identify ways to bring balance into your life.

What is one way to bring balance into your life?

The Life Balance Pyramid

IMMEDIATE COPING SKILLS

- Relax with deep breathing
- Use positive self-talk
- Envision a pleasant place

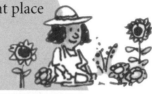

DAILY SUPPORTIVE ACTIVITIES

Pleasurable Activities
- Enjoy a warm bath
- Give and get hugs
- Laugh often

Physical Nourishment
- Be physically active
- Get plenty of rest
- Eat a variety of foods

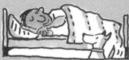

Social Connection
- Spend time with family, friends and pets
- Do kind deeds for others
- Volunteer time to a worthy cause

Emotional Well-being
- Nurture a positive self-image
- Express feelings in honest, fair, and direct ways
- Write in a journal

LIFELONG FOUNDATIONS

- Find fulfillment in hobbies or work
- Make time for meditation or prayer
- Connect with nature

- View life's challenges as opportunities
- Reflect on your personal values, goals, and choices
- Manage your diabetes

BUSH

C BUSH

When Life Gets in the Way

Managing diabetes can be particularly challenging when other problems intrude in your life. There are options to help you when you are having trouble with motivation or emotional issues.

Do you sometimes struggle with staying motivated? Maintaining motivation can be difficult when you are dealing with a disease that is life changing. You might find that your motivation changes a lot over time. Focus on giving yourself credit for all the things you do that keep you healthy and pay less attention to the things that are a struggle. Remember that you are in charge of your diabetes; it is not in charge of you.

Do you often feel negative, hopeless, or just numb? You may be struggling with depression. People with diabetes are nearly twice as likely to get depressed as others. When you no longer enjoy favorite activities or your mood is negative most of the time, consider talking to your care team about getting an emotional health assessment.

Do you often feel worried or afraid? You may have anxiety. Having a chronic illness (such as diabetes) may raise your risk of developing an anxiety problem. If left untreated, anxiety can interfere with many parts of life and is another good reason to get an emotional health assessment.

If you identify with any of these issues, your care team can recommend a professional who can evaluate your situation and suggest a number of treatment options (such as talking with a psychologist or social worker, taking medication, or both).

More on Healthy Eating

Fiber. Fiber is good for you. Eating more high-fiber foods can help with digestion, lower cholesterol, and may help you feel more full. Fiber is found in vegetables, fruits, whole grains, and dried beans. Try to eat at least five servings of vegetables and fruits every day. Choose other high-fiber foods such as cereals, breads, and crackers made from whole grains. Substituting beans for meat at some meals is another way to boost your fiber intake.

Fish. Certain fish contain omega-3 fatty acids, which are beneficial for your heart. These fatty acids help lower triglyceride levels. Eating two servings of fatty fish per week may reduce your heart disease risk. Lake trout, albacore tuna, salmon, herring, sardines, and mackerel are examples of fish that are high in omega-3 fatty acids. The body can also make omega-3 fatty acids from walnuts and flaxseed.

Dietary supplements. Many people with diabetes consider trying a dietary supplement like chromium or cinnamon to improve glucose levels. At this time, there isn't enough quality research to make a general recommendation for adding supplements. Some may not be safe or may interfere with other medications you are taking. Or they may not be the same from one brand or bottle to another. If you choose to try a supplement, follow these guidelines:

- Let your care team know if you are using a supplement.

- Only add one supplement at a time.

- Look for the "USP" verified mark. This tells you if the ingredients are accurate and pure.

- Only use the amount listed on the packaging (not more).

- Keep records to see if there is any improvement in your glucose level.

If you find there is no improvement in your glucose levels, consider stopping the supplement.

A Closer Look at Food Labels

Sugar-free or fat-free foods seem like they should be better food choices for people with diabetes. But this isn't always true.

Food labels help you uncover the real story. Read and compare the labels for regular, sugar-free, and fat-free cookies on the next page. Check the answers to the questions below.

1. Which has the most carbohydrate?

   ☐ Regular ☐ Sugar-free ☐ Fat-free ☐ All the same

2. Which has the most fat?

   ☐ Regular ☐ Sugar-free ☐ Fat-free ☐ All the same

3. Which has the most calories?

   ☐ Regular ☐ Sugar-free ☐ Fat-free ☐ All the same

4. Which cookie is the best?

   ☐ Oatmeal Raisin
   ☐ Fat-Free Oatmeal Raisin
   ☐ Sugar-Free Oatmeal

There isn't one right answer. The right choice for you is whichever cookie best matches your food plan goals.

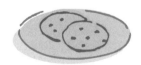

Oatmeal Raisin

Nutrition Facts

Serving Size 1 Cookie (26g)
Servings Per Container About 12

Amount Per Serving

Calories 110   Calories from Fat 30

	%Daily Value*
Total Fat 3.5g	5%
Saturated Fat 1g	4%
Cholesterol Less than 5mg	1%
Sodium 100mg	4%
Total Carbohydrate 17g	6%
Dietary Fiber 1g	3%
Sugars 9g	
Protein 1g	

Fat-Free Oatmeal Raisin

Nutrition Facts

Serving Size 1 Cookie (31g)
Servings Per Container About 10

Amount Per Serving

Calories 110   Calories from Fat 0

	%Daily Value*
Total Fat 0g	0%
Saturated Fat 0g	0%
Cholesterol 0mg	0%
Sodium 170mg	7%
Total Carbohydrate 25g	8%
Dietary Fiber 1g	4%
Sugars 14g	
Protein 1g	

Sugar-Free Oatmeal

Nutrition Facts

Serving Size 1 Cookie (24g)
Servings Per Container About 8

Amount Per Serving

Calories 110   Calories from Fat 45

	%Daily Value*
Total Fat 5g	8%
Saturated Fat 1g	6%
Cholesterol 0mg	0%
Sodium 75mg	3%
Total Carbohydrate 16g	5%
Dietary Fiber 0g	0%
Sugars 0g	
Protein 1g	

Choosing a Healthy Weight-Loss Plan

Losing just ten or fifteen pounds can improve your glucose, blood pressure, and cholesterol. If you are not sure how to choose a weight-loss plan, see the tips below.

Look for plans that ...	Be cautious about plans that ...
Focus on health	Focus on pounds
Aim for gradual, reasonable weight loss	Promise quick, significant weight loss
Promote a variety of foods in moderation	Ban entire food groups
Teach you how to include foods you like	Require you to eat only special foods or products
Encourage regular activity	Say activity isn't needed

Weight-loss medications are available. To be successful, they usually need to be taken long-term and combined with lifestyle changes. If your weight-loss needs are significant, surgery is also an option. Discuss your plan or concerns with your provider.

Weight-Loss Tips

- Start with clear and reasonable expectations.

- Eat breakfast. Studies show that it increases the likelihood of success.

- Remember that an occasional not-so-healthy food is OK.

- Recruit a friend and motivate each other.

- Participate in regular activity. This helps keep weight off.

- Keep a food and activity journal to track your progress.

Keeping Active

You've learned that activity helps with glucose control, lowers your resistance to insulin, and helps keep the heart healthy. Even so, one of the challenges to an active lifestyle is staying motivated. Busy lives have a way of getting in the way of even the best intentions.

Tips to Stay Active

- Ask a friend or spouse to join you.

- Make an appointment with yourself for physical activity (put it on your calendar).

- Build physical activity into your breaks and lunch hour.

- Have a plan for bad weather days.

- Share your activity goal with someone.

- Check the effect of activity on your glucose level.

Physical activity that builds muscle strength can also be helpful. This is achieved by doing repetitive exercises with weights, weight machines, or exercise bands. Before beginning this type of activity, check with your provider.

Research shows that people who combine heart healthy and strength training activity get more health benefits. It can also be a great combination for people trying to lose weight and keep it off.

Staying in Charge of Your Diabetes

Diabetes is a part of your life every day. Your provider will help you assess your glucose control and make changes as needed at your regular care visits. Together, you will also monitor your blood pressure, cholesterol, foot health, and other related health matters.

The more you know and understand about diabetes, the better you'll be able to manage it day to day. As time goes on, you will continue to learn and improve your skills.

It can be helpful to have a diabetes education tune-up each year. Depending on your individual needs, your care team may be able to direct you to:

- Support groups

- A psychologist or social worker

- Cooking classes

- Motivational resources

- Community education classes

- Fitness programs

If any of these are of interest to you, let your care team know.

Congratulations!

You've successfully completed Type 2 Diabetes BASICS. You've gained knowledge, skills, and tools to help you live healthfully with diabetes in the days, weeks, and months to come.

Your commitment to taking care of your diabetes is something to be proud of. Take time to congratulate yourself and to celebrate.

Remember, too, that your family and friends can be your strongest support system as you move on. Include them in your learning process. Share your experience of living well with diabetes.

Here's to you and to your health!

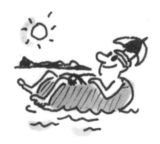

Appendix

Answer Key

Practice Carb Counting from page 25

Breakfast:	Orange juice	1	(15 grams)
	Cereal	2	(30 grams)
	Milk	1	(12 grams)
	Toast	1	(15 grams)
	Peanut butter	0	
	Banana	2	(30 grams)
	Total carb choices =	***7***	***(102 grams)***

Lunch or	Roast beef	0	
Evening Meal:	Baked potato	2	(30 grams)
	Green beans	0	
	Lettuce salad	0	
	w/Italian dressing	0	
	Dinner roll	1	(15 grams)
	Butter	0	
	Cookies	1	(15 grams)
	Coffee	0	
	Total carb choices =	***4***	***(60 grams)***

Snack:	Popcorn	2	(30 grams)
	Total carb choices =	***2***	***(30 grams)***

Fast-Food Meal:	Cheeseburger	2	(30 grams)
	French fries	3	(45 grams)
	Diet soft drink	0	
	Ice cream cone	1½	(22 grams)
	Total carb choices =	***6½***	***(97 grams)***

Food Label Quiz from page 26

Answers
1. 1 bar; 2. 6 servings; 3. 27 grams; 4. 2 choices

Heart Healthy Quick Check from page 83

How can you make these two meals more heart healthy?

Meal 1	Amount	Heart Healthy Choice
Prime rib	10 oz	6 oz tenderloin
Baked potato	6 oz (4-inches long)	(no change)
Butter	2 Tbsp	1 tsp tub margarine
Dinner salad	1 small	(no change)
French dressing, regular	2 Tbsp	1 Tbsp low-fat
Dinner roll	1 roll	(no change)
Butter	2 Tbsp	1 tsp tub margarine
Red wine	5 oz	(no change)

Meal 2	Amount	Heart Healthy Choice
Pasta	2 cups	1 cup
Meatballs	3	2
Tomato sauce	1 cup	½ cup
Soft bread stick	1 small	(no change)
Butter	1 Tbsp	1 tsp tub margarine
Dinner salad	1 small	(no change)
Italian dressing, regular	2 Tbsp	1 Tbsp low-fat
Milk, 2%	1 cup	skim or 1%

A Closer Look at Food Labels from page 98

Answers
1. Fat-free; 2. Sugar-free; 3. All the same; 4. There isn't one right answer.

107

Diabetes Medications

Diabetes Pills

Numerous pills are available to help treat diabetes. You can use some of these pills with insulin. Drug companies are making new types of diabetes pills all the time.

Sulfonylureas help your pancreas release more insulin.

Brand Name	Generic Name	Typical Dose
Amaryl®	Glimepiride	1–8 mg, 1 time daily with meal
Glucotrol®	Glipizide	2.5–20 mg, 1–2 times daily, 30 minutes before meals
Glucotrol XL®	Glipizide (extended release)	10 mg, 1 time daily with meal
DiaBeta® Micronase®	Glyburide	2.5–20 mg, 1–2 times daily with meals
Glynase®	Glyburide	1.5–6 mg, 1–2 times daily with meals

Meglitinides briefly help your pancreas make more insulin.

Brand Name	Generic Name	Typical Dose
Prandin®	Repaglinide	1–4 mg, 2–4 times daily with meals

D-phenylalanine derivate drugs briefly helps your pancreas make more insulin.

Brand Name	Generic Name	Typical Dose
Starlix®	Nateglinide	120 mg, up to 3 times daily with meals

Biguanides stop your liver from making extra glucose and help your body use insulin better.

Brand Name	Generic Name	Typical Dose
Glucophage®	Metformin	1,000 mg, 2 times daily with meals
Glucophage® XR	Metformin (extended release)	2,000 mg, 1 time daily with evening meal
Riomet®	Metformin oral solution	1,000 mg (10 mL), 2 times daily with meals
Glumetza®	Metformin extended release	2,000 mg, with evening meal

Thiazolidinediones makes muscle and fat cells more sensitive to insulin.

Brand Name	Generic Name	Typical Dose
Actos®	Pioglitazone	15–45 mg, 1 time daily
Avandia®	Rosiglitazone	4–8 mg, 1–2 times daily

Alpha-Glucosidase Inhibitors slow the body's absorption of carbohydrate.

Brand Name	Generic Name	Typical Dose
Precose®	Acarbose	25–100 mg, 3 times daily with meals
Glyset®	Miglitol	25–100 mg, 3 times daily with meals

Therapies for Incretin Deficiency help the pancreas cells work better.

Brand Name	Generic Name	Typical Dose
Januvia®	Sitagliptin	100 mg, 1 time daily
Onglyza®	Saxagliptin	2.5–5 mg, 1 time daily

Combination Pills contain two or more medicines in one pill. Many diabetes pills come in combination forms.

Other	Other Name	Typical Dose

Injectible Medications, Noninsulin help your pancreas cells work better and may help you eat less.

Brand Name	Generic Name	Typical Dose
Byetta®	Exenatide	5–10 mcg, 2 times daily up to one hour before meals
Victoza®	Liraglutide	1.2–1.8 mg, 1 time daily

Insulin Action Times

The table below shows how long each kind of insulin works after it's injected. The time when insulin is working hardest is called peak effect. After that, it works less and less, until it stops working.

Insulin (Brand name/generic name)	Starts Working	Works Hardest	Stops Working
BACKGROUND			
Long-acting Lantus® (glargine) Levemir® (detemir)	2 hrs	Steady most of the day*	Up to 24 hrs
Intermediate-acting **NPH** Humulin® N, Novolin® N	2–4 hrs	4–8 hrs	10–16 hrs
MEALTIME			
Rapid-acting Apidra® (glulisine) Humalog® (lispro) NovoLog® (aspart)	5–15 mins	1–2 hrs	3–4 hrs
Short-acting **Regular** Humulin® R, Novolin® R	30–45 mins	2–3 hrs	4–8 hrs
PREMIXED			
Intermediate-acting/rapid-acting Humalog® Mix 75/25 Humalog® Mix 50/50 (lispro protamine/lispro) NovoLog® Mix 70/30 (aspart protamine/aspart)	5–15 mins	1–2 hrs/some increase at 4–8 hrs	10–16 hrs
NPH/Regular Humulin® 70/30, Novolin® 70/30	30–45 mins	2–3 hrs/4–8 hrs	10–16 hrs

* In some people, long-acting insulins may work harder between 4 to 8 hours than the rest of the day.

Diabetes Care Schedule for Adults

Check Points	How Often	Goal
A1C	Every three to six months	Less than 7%
Blood pressure	Every three months	Less than 130/80 mmHg
LDL	Every year	Less than 100 mg/dL (with heart disease, less than 70 mg/dL)
HDL	Every year	Greater than 40 mg/dL (consider greater than 50 mg/dL for women)
Triglycerides	Every year	Less than 150 mg/dL
Urine protein as albumin-to-creatinine ratio	Every year	Less than 30 mg/g Cr
Aspirin use	Daily (if your provider recommends)	Ongoing
Retinal eye exam	Every year	Normal
Visual foot exam	Every three months	Normal
Complete foot exam	Every year	Normal
Dental exam	Every six months	Normal
Treatment plan review	Every three months	Ongoing
Diabetes education	Every year	Ongoing
Flu vaccine	Every year	
Pneumonia vaccine	Starting at age 65	

Healthy Snack Ideas

Snacks can fit into a healthy diet *if* good choices are made. The following snack choices listed contain about 15 grams of carb, 3 grams or less of saturated fat, and 250 mg or less of sodium. Look for brands that contain no trans fats. Add your favorite healthy snacks to the list.

Bread and Crackers

1 slice bread
2 slices light bread
½ small bagel or English muffin
1 small, low-fat muffin (1 oz)
9 Honey Maid® grahams honey sticks
4 RyKrisps®
6 reduced-fat Triscuits®
10 Kashi® TLC crackers
6 saltine crackers
10 reduced-fat Wheat Thins®
15 honey Teddy Grahams®
40 Goldfish® crackers
Other: _____

Fruit

1 small piece of fresh fruit
1 small banana (or ½ medium)
1 cup berries or melon
12–15 grapes or cherries
½ cup canned fruit in light syrup
1 miniature box of raisins (0.5 oz)
½ cup natural applesauce
Other: _____

Dairy

6 oz light, unsweetened,
  or plain yogurt
1 bottle Dannon Light & Fit™
  Smoothie
1 Jell-O® smoothie snack (4 oz)
Other: _____

Snack Foods

10–15 Baked Lays® potato chips
10 Baked Tostitos® tortilla chips
15 pretzel twists
3 cups microwave popcorn, light
¾ cup dry Cheerios®
½ cup dry Frosted Mini Wheats®
½ cup dry Quaker Oatmeal Squares®
Other: _____

Sweets

½ cup regular Jell-O®
1 frozen fruit bar
1 fudgsicle
½ cup frozen yogurt
½ cup light or low-fat ice cream
1 Rice Krispies Treat® 2" square
1 low-fat or Kashi® granola bar
5–6 vanilla wafers
3 gingersnaps
8 animal crackers
2 Snackwells® Crème Sandwich Cookies
3 Crème Savers® or other hard candies
Other: _____

Beverages

1 cup skim milk
½ cup orange or grapefruit juice
8 oz Diet V-8 Splash®
4 oz V-8 Splash®
1 packet no-sugar added cocoa
12 oz latte, with skim milk
12 oz cappuccino, with skim milk
Other: _____

Free Foods

The following snacks are considered *low-carb* and are *free* in the amounts listed below. These snacks have five or fewer grams of carb, less than 20 calories, and will not have a major effect on glucose levels.

Pickle, dill, 1 large
Popsicle, sugar-free, 1 stick
Salsa, ¼ cup
Vegetables, raw
Tomato/vegetable juice, ½ cup
Soft drinks, diet

Kool-Aid® or flavored drinks,
  sugar-free
Gelatin, sugar-free
Club soda
Tea, hot or iced, unsweetened

Low-Carb Snacks

The following snacks listed are *low-carb*. They also contain protein and fat. Although they have no major effect on glucose levels, they are higher in calories than free foods.

Eggs, hard-boiled, fried or
  scrambled
String cheese
Cottage cheese, ½ cup
Hummus
Omelet, all kinds
Olives, black or green, up to 15

Raw vegetables with ¼ cup dip
Celery, with 1 Tbsp peanut butter
Nuts:
  Almonds, 2 Tbsp
  Peanuts, in shell, ½ cup
  Peanuts, no shells, 2 Tbsp
  Sunflower seeds, in shells,
    ½ cup

Dining Out Favorites

	Carb Grams	Carb Choices	Fat Grams
Breakfast Foods			
Bagel, large (most bagel shops)	60–75	4–5	2–7
Breakfast sandwich, English muffin	27	2	12
Donut, cake (plain or frosted), 3"	27–36	2–2½	12–19
Muffin, jumbo	60–85	4–5½	10–35
Soups/Chili			
Chili, with meat and beans, 1 cup	24–27	1½–2	6–10
Sandwiches/Burgers			
Bagel sandwich	60–75	4–5	4–50
Burger, fast food or restaurant, ¼ lb, with bun and mayo or sauce	37–47	2½–3	19–41
Fish sandwich, breaded	41–59	3–4	14–31
Roast beef sandwich, fast-food	26–33	2	10–19
Sub sandwich, 6"	41–48	3	3–21
Salads			
Taco salad, no shell, with toppings, large	14–25	1–1½	19–25
Asian Entrees			
Chow mein, beef or chicken, no rice or noodles, 1 cup	17–24	1–1½	6–20
Chow mein noodles, crispy, ½ cup	13	1	7
Egg roll, 5"	23	1½	5–11
Lo mein, meat or vegetable, 1 cup	35–47	2–3	11–17
Rice, fried, 1 cup	42–52	3–3½	10–16
Stir fry, with meat, no rice or noodles, 1 cup	16	1	4–10
Sweet-and-sour chicken or pork, no rice or noodles, 1½ cups	43–53	3–3½	25–35
Indian Entrees			
Chapati or Roti, 7"	11	1	0.5
Naan, 8"x 2"	11	1	2
Dal (dhal), ½ cup	18	1	0.5

	Carb Grams	Carb Choices	Fat Grams
Italian Entrees			
Fettuccine Alfredo, 1½ cups	58–64	4	13–30
Lasagna, with meat, 3½" square	68	4½	41
Parmigiana, chicken or veal, no sauce or pasta	5–13	0–1	20
Mexican Entrees			
Burrito, 6"	47–58	3–4	7–36
Enchilada, with cheese and meat, 4"	18–31	1–2	6–19
Quesadilla, 8–10"	30–41	2–3	18–31
Taco, soft shell, fast-food, 6"	16–27	1–2	8–14
Pizza*			
Pizza, personal (6"), 1 whole	68–71	4½–5	22–50
Pizza, thick crust, medium (12–14"), ⅛ pizza	27–40	2–2½	6–15
Pizza, thin crust, medium (12–14"), ⅛ pizza	19–22	1–1½	6–11
* For a very thin crust, use lower number in the range; for a super thick crust, use the higher number.			
Side Dishes			
Potato, baked, with skin and toppings, 4–5"	44–56	3–4	6–12
Snacks			
Nachos, with cheese, large or thick chips, 6–8	27–43	2–3	19–23
Desserts and Sweets			
Cheesecake, plain, ¹⁄₁₂ of 9" cake	36–44	2½–3	25–37
Ice cream, premium, ½ cup	20–34	1–2	15–24
Pie, fruit, ⅙ of 8" pie	56–73	4–5	19–37
Pie, pumpkin or custard, ⅙ of 8" pie	38	2½	7

Fat content varies due to differences in preparation. For those trying to watch their weight or cholesterol, one fat serving equals 5 grams of fat.

Sweeteners

Sugars and sugar substitutes sweeten foods. Some of them affect glucose levels, while others don't.

Nutrition Facts	
Serving Size 1 Bar (34g)	
Servings Per Container 1 Bar	

Amount Per Serving	
Calories 140	Calories from Fat 70
	% Daily Value*
Total Fat 7g	**11%**
Saturated Fat 3.5g	**18%**
Trans Fat 0g	
Cholesterol 5mg	**2%**
Sodium 70mg	**3%**
Total Carbohydrate 24g	**5%**
Dietary Fiber 3g	**20%**
Sugars 10g	
Sugar Alcohol 8g	
Protein 4g	

Sugars

Sugar comes in many forms. Examples include table sugar, honey, brown sugar, and pancake syrup. Count sugars as carbohydrates in your food plan.

- 1 level Tbsp sugar (all types) = 1 carb choice or 15 grams of carb

Sugar Substitutes or Artificial Sweeteners

Sugar substitutes and artificial sweeteners are very low in carbs and calories, so they are "free" (you don't need to count them). They will not affect your glucose levels. Check with the manufacturer before cooking with sugar substitutes. Some require special recipes or may not remain sweet if heated. Used in moderation, they are safe. Examples include:

Aspartame (NutraSweet®)   Acesulfame K (Sweet One®)
Sucralose (Splenda®)   Saccharin (Sweet'N Low®)

Sugar Alcohols

Sugar alcohols are found in many products marked *sugar-free*. They are carbs, but the body doesn't completely absorb them. This means they have less affect on glucose levels than sugar. Sugar alcohols are included on the *Nutrition Facts* food label under "Total Carbohydrate." If more than 5 grams, subtract half of the sugar alcohol grams from the total amount of carb listed. Some people experience a laxative effect when eating foods with sugar alcohols. Examples include sorbitol and manitol.

Sample Menus

Menus for Women Who Want to Lose Weight

Breakfast
1 slice whole-wheat toast
soft margarine
⅓ melon
coffee

Breakfast
small vegetable omelet
1 slice toast
soft margarine
2 small plums
tea

Lunch
1 cup chicken vegetable soup
½ turkey sandwich
    (1 slice whole-wheat bread)
1 orange
ice water

Lunch
1 low-calorie frozen dinner
tossed salad, light dressing
diet soft drink

Evening meal
grilled fish
1 small baked potato
broccoli
low-fat sour cream
1 cup strawberries
1 cup low-fat milk

Evening meal
1 cup casserole
1 cup green beans
1 cup skim milk

Each menu has 2–3 carb choices per meal; 30–45 grams of carb (about 1,200 calories*).

* To stay close to this calorie level, assumes low-fat cooking methods, light or low-fat food choices when possible, small portions of added fats, and two to three ounces of cooked meat or other protein at a meal (about the size of a deck of cards).

Menus for Men Who Want to Lose Weight or Women Who Want to Maintain Weight

Breakfast
1 cup oatmeal
1 cup low-fat milk
coffee

Breakfast
1 English muffin
soft margarine
1 cup light yogurt
peanut butter
tea

Lunch
1 cup chili
6 saltine crackers
sugar-free gelatin
1 cup melon
carrot and celery sticks
sugar-free lemonade

Lunch
grilled chicken sandwich
  (2 slices bread)
1 cup low-fat cabbage salad
1 small apple
1 cup low-fat milk

Evening meal
2 pieces vegetable pizza
1 small fresh fruit
1 medium cookie
1 diet soft drink

Evening meal
1½ cups casserole
tossed salad, light dressing
1 small dinner roll
1 diet soft drink

Each menu has 3–4 carb choices per meal; 45–60 grams of carb (about 1,500 calories*).

* To stay close to this calorie level, assumes low-fat cooking methods, light or low-fat food choices when possible, small portions of added fats, and two to three ounces of cooked meat or other protein at a meal (about the size of a deck of cards).

Menus for Men Who Want to Maintain Weight

Breakfast
3 pancakes (6" across)
Canadian bacon
sugar-free pancake syrup
soft margarine
½ cup orange juice
coffee

Breakfast
1½ cup dry cereal
1 cup 1% milk
1 slice toast
soft margarine
tea

Lunch
sandwich (2 slices bread)
tossed salad, light dressing
1 small apple
2 small cookies
1 cup skim milk

Lunch
large fast-food hamburger
small French fries
diet soft drink

Evening meal
1½ cups chicken stir-fry
1 cup rice
1 fortune cookie
tea

Evening meal
4 oz steak
1 medium baked potato with
    light sour cream
1 dinner roll
tossed salad, light dressing
12–15 grapes
1 cup low-fat milk

Each menu has 4–5 carb choices; 60–75 grams of carb (about 1,800 calories*).

* To stay close to this calorie level, assumes low-fat cooking methods, light or low-fat food choices when possible, small portions of added fats, and two to four ounces of cooked meat or other protein at a meal (about the size of a deck of cards).